Locker Room Diaries

Locker Room Diaries

*The Naked Truth About Women,
Body Image, and Re-Imagining the "Perfect" Body*

LESLIE GOLDMAN

Da Capo

**LIFE
LONG**

A Member of the Perseus Books Group

Designed by Trish Wilkinson
Set in 11-point Garamond by The Perseus Books Group

Library of Congress Cataloging-in-Publication Data

Goldman, Leslie.
    Locker room diaries : the naked truth about women, body image, and re-imagining the "perfect" body / Leslie Goldman. — 1st Da Capo Press ed.
        p.   cm.
    ISBN-13: 978-0-7382-1042-1 (hardcover : alk. paper)
    ISBN-10: 0-7382-1042-0 (hardcover : alk. paper) 1. Women—Psychology. 2. Body image in women. 3. Self-esteem in women. 4. Nudity— Psychological aspects. 5. Physical fitness centers—Social aspects. I. Title.
HQ1206.G723 2006
306.4—dc22   2006009059

Published by Da Capo Press
A Member of the Perseus Books Group
http://www.dacapopress.com

Da Capo Press books are available at special discounts for bulk purchases in the U.S. by corporations, institutions, and other organizations. For more information, please contact the Special Markets Department at the Perseus Books Group, 11 Cambridge Center, Cambridge, MA 02142, or call (800) 255-1514 or (617) 252-5298, or email special.markets@perseusbooks.com.

1 2 3 4 5 6 7 8 9—09 08 07 06

For Dan,
whose insight has been invaluable;
his love and support, unparalleled

It's in the arch of my back,
The sun of my smile,
The ride of my breasts,
The grace of my style.
I'm a woman
Phenomenally.
Phenomenal woman,
That's me.

—Maya Angelou

Contents

So I tried on my wedding dress last night.
The back and arms need serious work.

—Woman in her early thirties to trainer,
overheard in locker room

I wish I could just slice off this part of my thigh, from
here to here. That would be perfect.

—Woman in her mid-twenties to a girlfriend,
overheard in locker room

Honey, let's get on the scale and
see if you've lost anything.

—Mother to young daughter, approximately
ten years old, overheard in locker room

Introduction:
Warming Up

When I learned Crunch Fitness had installed peekaboo showers in their locker rooms, enticing members to watch their fellow gym-goers soap up from behind silhouetted glass doors, I was amused and, admittedly, a bit intrigued.

When 24 Hour Fitness launched a billboard campaign featuring an alien along with the proclamation, "When they come, they'll eat the fat ones first," I was horribly disturbed.

But when I discovered Women's Workout World had a "No Nudity" policy in their club's locker rooms, I was blown away.

"We deal with women from all walks of life, all different shapes, cultures, and religions," explained CEO Shari Whitley. The "No Nudity" policy, she believes, fosters a nonthreatening atmosphere, one that especially helps women who have issues with body image.

So there it was: Women's self-esteem has become so needy that although some of us feel it necessary to perform a wet burlesque show for the weight room while we shower

("Oops, I dropped the soap!"), others are so fragile that "No Nudity" clauses are now needed . . . *in locker rooms.* I knew something had to be done.

That's why in the time it takes to read this introduction, I'll likely have witnessed more naked women up close and personal than the average adult male sees in his lifetime. Yes, from gazing at gazongas to poring over pedicures, for the past few years I have immersed myself in the locker room of my gym, scribbling notes, eavesdropping, stealing glances, and, when the situation called for it, just downright, blatantly staring. Some might call this sort of behavior rude—invasive, even. I call it research.

What I conducted, essentially, is an ethnography of the ladies' locker room (and in the process I raised more than a few male friends' and colleagues' eyebrows). It began innocently enough: I was just starting graduate school, earning my master's degree in public health with a focus on women's health. Having grown up in the impenetrable bubble of northwestern suburban Chicago, where taking a baseball bat to a mailbox is cause for a town-hall meeting, I was new to the city and needed to join a gym. A nice, safe gym—my only requirement being that men did not lift weights in cut-off jeans and construction boots. Did such a thing exist?

I found a great place, a relatively expensive health club with all the amenities: from disposable razors, lotion, and mouthwash to an onsite manicurist and Reiki healer. I mean, there was even a rooftop sundeck with a tiki hut and bar.

But for me, the real action was in the locker room. Within my first few days of working out, I started to take note of the insults women hurled at themselves like drunken Cubs fans, the public trading of body flaws like so many stocks and bonds. In what began as a sort of informal thesis, I started carrying my faux leopard fur-covered journal in my gym bag. Every day in that locker room, I would scribble down what I saw and heard. And in a culture where women are essentially trained to loathe their bodies, it wasn't long before I had a diary chock-full of anecdotes and stories—some of them disheartening, some inspiring, but all poignant.

Take, for instance, the attractive, slim twenty-something woman who approached me from behind as I applied my lipstick one evening. She wore a silver two-piece bathing suit, apparently ready to hit the hot tub. As she walked closer and closer, I eyed her toned physique through the mirror and felt a twinge of envy. Just as the thought, "I wish I looked like that in a metallic string bikini," traveled through my head, the woman slapped her thighs and shouted out in disgust, to nobody in particular, "Ugh—I'm so FAT!"

Was she searching for some sort of sick camaraderie from me? Or was this self-deprecating comment merely rhetorical? Regardless, the message was clear: This woman hated her body, imaginary flaws and all.

From the women with immaculate physiques who change in the bathroom stalls to avoid imagined public scrutiny to the heavier women who stroll around naked without a care in the world; from the women who wax everything—and I do mean *everything*—to women who shave down south only for their yearly gynecological exam; from breast implants and mastectomy scars to bellies swollen from pregnancy and asses sagging from old age, every body part and every owner has a story to tell—and a lesson we can learn.

When we are naked, we are at our most vulnerable—physically and emotionally. When we are naked, there are no Miracle bras to lift our 34Bs to magnificent heights, no control-top panty hose to smooth away the dimples, no high heels to coax our calf muscles out of hiding. Without the armor of clothing, we fall prey much more easily to low self-esteem, personal insecurities, and the scrutiny of those around us. Like animals in the wild, we are in our bare, natural state, with nothing to hide us except a measly rectangular strip of towel. Skin hangs and wobbles, blemishes emerge, hair sprouts from places we didn't know it could grow. Ah, yes, fluorescent lighting. From the self-deprecating comments I continue to hear uttered by and between women, the bodily obsessions and emotional vulnerability reflected in the mirror and on the scale, I have come to realize that the locker room is where women literally let it all hang out. Beneath the unforgiving lights and amongst the stolen glances from fellow females, I've gained a new understanding for how what goes on in the women's locker room can be viewed as a distillation of our body-obsessed society's impact on women.

I believe it's time we tame the disparaging inner demon that paralyzes so many women into a state of broken body image and delve deeper into the question of why—why have we succumbed to this culture-induced cacophony of "if-onlys"? *If only* I could be thinner. *If only* my breasts could be as firm as hers. *If only* my ass could be that high. *If only* I could be that sexy. That curvy. That waif-like. The adjective doesn't even matter, so long as the grass is greener (and neatly trimmed into a Brazilian bikini landscape). Though these locker room lessons—whether about growing older, giving birth, getting cancer, or braving therapy—may differ, the ultimate maxim will emerge universal: Slay the demon, screw the scale, and live large, no matter what you weigh.

Through my (mis)adventures, the locker room has become my second home. It's where I shower and shave, gossip and gab. I venture to my gym five, even six times a week. (Although sometimes exercise isn't even required: I've been known to indulge in an occasional "executive workout"—a sauna and a shower—just to get my fix.) After each sweat-soaked, soul-cleansing workout, the locker room is my retreat. Inside, I and scores of other women peel off our clammy sports bras and strip down to our skivvies, our tired bodies begging for a warm shower and perhaps a reprieve from self-reproach.

But much more than that, the locker room is where I have learned about body image, the female form and the various neuroses that afflict it—more than any college anatomy class or well-worn therapist's couch has taught me. Time after time, I have listened as women chastise themselves and trade insults with girlfriends, sisters, or even their children, uttering the sorts of statements that would be deemed mentally abusive if a man were to spew them to his wife.

Having watched too many friends battle anorexia, bulimia, and compulsive exercising, I have seen the ways poor body image can wreak havoc on a young woman's physical and mental health. They are just a few of the eight million American women who struggle with a diagnosable eating disorder, according to the National Association of Anorexia Nervosa and Associated Disorders—and that number does not account for the untold others with disordered eating and distorted body image ("body image" referring to the way a woman perceives her physical appearance, as well as how she thinks others see her).

I was one of those women, too. For years, I struggled with an eating disorder—anorexia—that demolished my self-esteem during my first year of college faster than any unrequited freshman crush could ever have. I shed 30 pounds from my already slender five-foot-eleven frame before winter break through a diet of salsa-topped salad and seemingly endless nighttime runs across the University of Wisconsin–Madison's beautiful, sprawling campus. My face grew gaunt; my clothes hung from my skeletal frame as if from a hanger. All around me, chaos ensued—"What should we do with her? Why did this happen?" Meanwhile, I was busy hammering out my daily caloric intake on my calculator. I just didn't get it. I mean, five foot eleven and 120 pounds—that's what models weigh, right?

In a sad bit of irony, I was majoring in—and acing—nutritional sciences.

I am now considered recovered in terms of my eating disorder, meaning I don't actively engage in the destructive behaviors that overpowered me for so many years. Through a treatment regimen that consisted, at different times, of a variety of therapies and medications, I exorcised the demons that drove my pulse to 36 and my periods to a halt. But the inner critic will always remain and I, along with millions of otherwise successful women, continue to struggle with body image on some level.

From the constant trips to my university's drab public fitness facility to the high-gloss shine of my current health club, I've pretty much seen it all—and I suspect I'm not alone. According to the International Health, Racquet & Sportsclub Association, in 2004 (the latest year for which figures are available), 21.6 million American women had health club memberships.

This book is for any woman who has ever experienced the terror of stepping on a scale large enough for the entire locker room to read, or gotten tangled in a wet bathing suit when all she wanted was to be cloaked in a bathrobe, or desperately grasped at her towel as it slipped from her nude body, *just* as another woman walked behind her. It's for any woman who knows what the physical high of a great workout feels like, but continues to beat herself up emotionally. For any woman who has ever looked at another woman's breasts, hips, or stomach and wondered, "How do I compare to her?" (Remember the *Sex and the City* episode in which the famous foursome meet at a day spa for some R&R, only to learn that Charlotte is unable to shed her towel in the steam room, convinced other women are staring at her thighs?)

Considering the society we live in, is it any wonder I've found myself comparing cellulite with total strangers? Or looked on with envy as preteen girls enjoy the blossoming of their breasts while their hips remain narrow?

For years, these locker room observations and comments from the scores of women involved in this book have been marinating in my mind. We have spent far too many hours worrying about our bodies, how they look in the mirror, in our minds, and in other people's eyes. Let's take back time and reclaim some of those hours—if not for ourselves, then for the millions of other women who have struggled alongside us.

I remember, for instance, making my way to the showers one morning after a killer workout when something blonde and odd-shaped lying on the floor caught my eye: a wig. On my way back to my locker after lotioning up, I instinctively looked down to where the wig had lain, only to find an empty space. Now, it was atop the head of a beautiful, thirty-something woman dressed in business attire and applying her makeup. I later learned the young woman had lost her hair during treatment for breast cancer, which got me thinking about the importance we, as a society, place on physical looks, even in the midst of a potentially life-threatening disease.

It also filled me with admiration for her strength and vigor in continuing to exercise her way through cancer. I recall thinking, "I'd love to talk to her and learn from her." I since have and her story truly is awe inspiring.

Laura Berman, PhD, the famous sex therapist, calls distorted body image "an epidemic, affecting all parts of women's lives; in particular, their sex lives, but also how many outfits they try on in the morning before work, their sense of self-consciousness during the day, their self-esteem and their general quality of life."

"The fact is," she continues, "women in general look at each other and compare themselves—on the street, in the office, in the entertainment industry and in the locker room." It's at the point where fields such as genital rejuvenation (read: surgery or lasers) exist to answer the call of women fearful that their vaginas, let alone their stomachs or derrieres, don't measure up.

Further ingraining the notion of physical perfection and feeding women's starving body images are the recent reality television programs that chronicle women's (and men's) quests for physical perfection via tummy tucks, liposuction, breast lifts, porcelain veneers, nose jobs, and so forth. Even Lisa Simpson—yes, the cartoon—struggled with an eating disorder, as has her voice, Yeardley Smith. (Lisa's problem was solved within a thirty-minute episode, but Smith's battle with bulimia lasted more than a decade.) More extreme, another network premiered a sitcom . . . a *sitcom!* . . . called *Starved,* which followed four thirty-something friends, all of whom suffered from eating disorders. There was no laugh track.

Women also continue to be exposed to advertising that promotes an unattainable ideal, made all the more obvious beneath the glaring lights of the locker room. As Jean Kilbourne, EdD, the former model and advertising guru, once told me, "I've heard that even Cindy Crawford has said, 'I wish *I* looked like Cindy Crawford.'" In the three thousand or so advertisements we take in each day, women are typically airbrushed out of reality, with only a long, lean torso shown here, or a perfectly smooth rear-end displayed there. These images engender in women the feeling that our bodies are, and will always be, less-than, interchangeable, and somehow incomplete.

It both scares and deeply saddens me to imagine the hours, the days, indeed, the *years,* that my female counterparts and I have flushed down the toilet (often literally) thinking about which parts of our bodies we wish we could shave away, what we should eat for our next meal, how many calories we need to burn to cancel out last night's chocolate cake. I suspect that with my background in science I could have helped discover cures for both cancer and cellulite in the time I've spent agonizing over such meaningless inner dialogue.

That's why I'm ready for my fuzzy little notebook, a true labor of love and self-exploration, to go public.

And let's not forget the lesson learned by Charlotte from that locker room episode of *Sex and the City.* After her confidence is bolstered by a body-image pep talk with Carrie, Charlotte returns to the spa, tip-toeing through the locker room. She pauses nervously to unwrap her towel, enters the steam room, and bares all. Just as her nervousness is about to reach a fever pitch, validation comes in the form of another woman's voice: "I'd kill for your breasts."

1

Conquering Mount Toledo
Putting the Scale in Its Place

The scale in my gym's locker room is gargantuan, hideously oversized, like something you'd find in *Alice in Wonderland*. It lurks in the far back corner of the locker room, a menacing, six-foot-tall beast of a Toledo. It's the kind of scale found at fairs; only a brave man would dare climb it as a challenge to the carnival barker to guess his weight so that he can win his lady a stuffed animal. Gunmetal gray, it has a two-foot-by-two-foot rubber platform and a huge round register. When you step on it, the slender blood-red needle slowly rises like a psychological odometer, bobbing back and forth for a few excruciating seconds as it deliberates its final sentence.

Nearly every day for five years, I have watched—and, admittedly, joined—women as they prepared to climb this scale, almost all of us programmed with an eerily similar routine.

It begins when a woman of any given size or shape approaches the steely monster. Typically she is clad in just a towel and flip-flops. Actual clothing? Forget it. And shoes? Out of the question. What are you trying to do, *add* two pounds?

After a quick scan of the room to see whether anyone is nearby, the woman turns back and attempts to scale Mount Toledo. Stepping onto the platform, she takes a deep breath, imperceptible to all but the most attuned of gym-goers, and gazes up at the numbers, her eyes at once hopeful and dreading. The needle eventually settles, and one of two scenarios ensues.

If the number is favorable, she immediately hops off, as if hot coals were underfoot, just in case the needle is feeling fickle and decides to creep up a few more increments. Off she struts, as satisfied as if she were just on the receiving end of a one-hour massage—happy ending included.

But more often than not, the number is a disappointment. The woman is launched into a sort of weight-loss striptease— and I don't mean the kind Carmen Electra might perform. First, she untucks the corner of the white towel from beneath her arm and lets it slip to the ground. That shaves off another pound, especially if it's wet. Next, her flip-flops might be kicked away; then her wristwatch goes, placed atop the nearby pay phone. Another ounce or two. After that, with nothing else to remove, the woman stands there, naked, soaking in the final number and what it all-too-often represents: her self-worth.

It's just as my friend Debbie said to me one morning as she came into work: "I decided to be mean to myself this morning, so I got on the scale."

Drop the Towel and Slowly Step Away from the Scale

I have participated in this ritual many, many times. The frequency ebbs and flows, most recently flaring up prior to my wedding a few years ago. But for a good couple of years, I abstained. And here's why: One morning as I changed clothes, I heard the joyful voice of a young girl, maybe three years old. She was galloping around the locker room, playing peekaboo from behind the locker doors, blowing warm air from the hair dryers into her face, and generally just admiring herself in the mirrors. As her attention focused on the scale, I saw her climb up onto it with Herculean effort. She began to jump up and down, yelling for her mom to come see her in her newly conquered territory.

The mother followed her daughter's gleeful voice to The Scale, where she rumpled her daughter's hair, giving her a cursory "That's great, honey!" She lifted her daughter off the scale and then got on herself. In one swift motion, the mother's face soured and her head dropped. She stepped gingerly off the scale and, without another word, returned to her locker and continued dressing. And wouldn't you know it, before I had the chance to ask myself, "Will this turn into a vicious, lifelong cycle?" that little girl climbed back onto the scale and, in a performance worthy of a pint-sized Oscar, imitated her mother's actions, right down to her exaggerated pouty face. Was she old enough to read the numbers? Probably not. Did she even know what a scale was? I'd assume no. But in less than one minute, she had learned a lesson that would likely follow her the rest of her life: The scale is something that makes women sad.

I'll admit, for years—before, during, and for sometime after my eating disorder—I was a scale junkie. It was my crack, my smack, my fix. I'd jump on pretty much anything with a dial, be it in a locker room, in a friend's washroom, or at the doctor's office. I believe I once tried weighing myself in a sporting-goods store but chickened out. That number ruled my day.

What the hell was I thinking? First, let's ignore that, like fingerprints or taste in men, every scale is different, and they yield wildly dissimilar readouts. Next, disregard the fact that the average woman's weight can fluctuate by up to 5 pounds in one day, potentially leaving me as happy as the winner of a Tiffany & Co. shopping spree or as devastated as the runner up who gets the little horseshoe-shaped key chain with the screw-on balls.

But I swear on my dog-eared copy of *Reviving Ophelia,* the day I saw that little girl's unblemished body image tainted before my eyes as her mother scowled at Mount Toledo's reading, I changed my tune completely. My scale-hopping scaled back immediately, to the point where I refused to allow the nurse to weigh me during my annual physical exam (and still do). That little girl—and the power that I, as a grown woman, had over her and others like her—haunted me. It was a responsibility that I, as a young feminist concerned with the emotional and physical health of the next generation of women, felt tingling deep in my bones. Today, I continue to see young girls look on as everyone from pre-teens to older women climb the scale and succumb, or rise up, to the number. Always, I can read their minds. Not wanting to perpetuate that ritual, I stay away, hoping that they will also see me, a young, healthy woman, *not* stepping on the scale and *not* allowing the number to reign over my parade.

Of course, it would be a lie to say that I never weigh myself these days. Granted, I try to go by the scale of my figure rather than the figure on the scale. But a few times a year I find myself wondering, and I retreat to the back of the locker room. One of the lessons I've learned, however—besides absolutely never weighing myself when there are children around—is to do it quickly, minus the ritualistic dance of untucking my towel and discarding all accessories. Not because I'm afraid the number will be scary or will have the same hold on me it once had, but because I never again want to possess that look of desperation so many of my fellow gymgoers display on that funhouse platform.

Why have we intelligent women granted authority to this evil hunk of metal, not only over our bodies but over our minds? Only a good night's sleep, early-morning sex, or a nice vanilla latte should be allowed to wield so much influence over how we start our day. We should be as diligent about avoiding our locker room's scale as we are about ignoring catcalling construction workers whooping it up as we walk by.

And please, don't keep a scale in your home bathroom. The whole scenario is akin to that of an alcoholic who lives above a wine bar. Why don't you just go for a nice five-mile jog in your Jimmy Choos while you're at it?

David vs. Goliath

It's truly, sadly amazing that we women allow a scale to have such power over us—especially when there are so many other more worthwhile appliances to become reliant upon. Why not get hooked on our iPods? Our espresso machines? Our vibrators, yearning to be set free? All these modern conveniences make life so much easier, make our bodies feel so good, and yet we look to the scale for affirmation. One fellow Chicago author and gym-goer embroiled in her own weight loss battle, Erin, twenty-nine, calls the scale "a mindfuck"; another weight-loss blogger refers to herself as a "scale whore." It's a never-ending battle, one that won't stop until we topple all scales, like the crumbling of the Berlin Wall.

I have actually seen women stand in line, waiting to step on the scale in my locker room. You stand in line at Banana Republic, not at the scale! These women hang back patiently while those in front of them unlace their shoes, strip out of their sports bras, take off their jewelry. Some peer around for the readout, attempting to be subtle in their comparisons. No matter whether the physique standing before them is six inches taller or six inches shorter, smaller-boned or more athletic, pear- or apple-shaped—the number on the scale is all that matters.

At one point, when a woman standing four foot eleven and weighing 105 pounds stepped on the scale before me, I would fantasize, "Wouldn't it be great to be so petite?" But forty-eight hours later, if a 150-pound athletic swimmer with amazing definition in her back and shoulders stood on that register, I'd think, "Why don't I have muscles like that?"

One morning while observing women in the locker room, I ran into Sangeeta, thirty-eight, a law student I know from a weightlifting class at the gym. Sangeeta and I had bumped into each other just days earlier at a coffee shop, where I had told her a bit about my locker room ethnography and had asked her whether she had issues with the scale. Sangeeta said that although she hates weighing herself, she often feels compelled to do so, and she has a range she tries to stay within: At 114 pounds, she feels thin and happy; at 118, she feels uncomfortably heavy. To look at her, this seems silly—the woman is lithe but muscular, her caramel skin is smooth, her hair long and black. At five foot three, she somehow seems at least a few inches taller. Her body is fit and beautiful.

That morning in the locker room, Sangeeta had spotted me and was reminded of our coffee shop conversation. This, apparently, prompted her to hop on the scale. When I saw her a few minutes later, buttoning her khakis and pulling on her blouse, she smiled hello and then, scrunching up her nose (the only seemingly scrunchable part on her solid body), she said, "Today is a 118 day."

For a moment, I was confused—until she explained, "Remember our talk? At 114 pounds, I feel good. At 118, I feel fat." Then she looked me up and down—I was wearing a fleece and running pants—and commented, "You're so thin."

"No!" I thought. "This isn't supposed to be happening. This is the *opposite* of what's supposed to be happening. This is a *feel good* project, not some evil experiment in envy and comparison." I felt a bit dizzy and, admittedly, guilty. I gathered up my journal hidden inside a decoy magazine and ducked out pronto.

Why do we feel compelled to judge ourselves against others? Every woman has something to be proud of, be it powerful quads that can propel her across the tennis court, the kind of flexibility that even a yoga instructor covets, or the ability to jog on the treadmill while reading a magazine. Our fellow locker mates are not the enemy. The scale should not be the enemy. Ben and Jerry's New York Triple Fudge Chunk isn't even the enemy. The enemy lives within us. Let's start exorcising.

Just Say No

The celebrity trainer Kacy Duke has sculpted the biceps and tightened the tushes of such A-list stars as Kirsten Dunst,

Denzel Washington, Julianne Moore, and Lenny Kravitz. But she doesn't know how much they weigh. That's because the high-paced, hard-bodied Duke, who splits her time between New York and Los Angeles, shuns the scale. As creative director for the swanky Equinox gym chain, Duke spends more than her fair share of time in the locker room, where she has witnessed scale-induced frenzies of boy-band concert proportions.

She recalled one scene in particular: "I was in the locker room and this one woman who I thought had a pretty nice body got on the scale and started screaming, 'What am I working out this hard for?!' She couldn't see the forest for the trees." Women nearby, Duke confirmed, were actually chuckling to each other, clucking, "Crazy bitch. I'd die for her body." Meanwhile, this lady was having a conniption fit over what was likely a lower-than-average weight for her height.

But it's what happened next that warmed Duke's heart: Just minutes later, a woman on the heavier side who had recently begun working out stepped on the scale. She must have been satisfied with the number because, Duke remembered, she shouted out, "Yes!" (The way she recounts the story, I can only imagine that a fist pump accompanied the declaration.)

"I felt like it was God in action," Duke recalled, "telling me to look at this and remember. It was such a view of what's really important."

(Now, of course, this is a chapter about ditching the scale, about stopping the practice of looking to the dial as a source of confidence and affirmation. But the scenario Duke described is poignant because it shows how differently two women can react to a simple number and how, for an overweight woman on the pathway to health, that number represents success. So long as she doesn't get hooked, all is well.)

For Duke, what's really important is enjoying the *fitness journey* rather than focusing on a number on the scale. Her mantra: "Fitness is an evolution, not a revolution." If getting in shape is a journey, the scale is a roadblock. In her fairy tale–like description, "The scale becomes the Emerald City and you can't enjoy the yellow brick road."

So yes, she hates seeing scales in the locker room. She's even asked to have them removed, but management tells her that members demand them. When the scale in the women's locker room is broken, she said, frantic notes overflow from the suggestion box: "The scale is broken" and "Please fix the scale."

My friend Ali, thirty, brought this point home the other day when she told me she had gone to the gym to work out and weigh herself, only to find an "Out of order" sign hanging from the scale's neck. "I was so confused," she said. "It reminded me of the time I went to Starbucks and they told me they were out of coffee."

But although Ali's weight obsessions have fluctuated like those of most women, she's been able to keep her fixations in check—even through the often obsessive processes of training for a marathon and giving birth to a baby girl (as well as the accompanying weight gain, although she somehow managed not to show until her ninth month by carrying little Milla entirely inside her abdominal cavity). She doesn't weigh herself *that* often, maybe less than once a month. She and her husband don't even keep a scale in the house.

I asked Duke what, given the opportunity, she would say to that woman with the fabulous body who stepped on the scale only to start screaming and hollering about her "weight problem." Here's what she had to say:

> I would ask her to walk around the park with me and ask her to see what I see. To see a man with only one leg running, or an older woman walking, just for the health of it. To see how important it is that she has a life and that she should live it to the fullest, not just for the physical aspects. It's about being really healthy and fit and doing something that says, "I'm alive." Fitness is like great sex—it's an amazing thing. It makes you feel so lucky to be moving and living. Why get bogged down by the scale?

The Abstainers

Why get bogged down, indeed. In the course of researching this book, I came across a rare breed of women who never weigh themselves. I mean, they never, ever weigh themselves. I had originally thought this group was indigenous to sub-Saharan tribes where scales don't exist; but no, these are real American women, purposely choosing to eschew the scale. Quite often, it seems, they have had eating issues in the past, and so they avoid the scale because, as Duke said, it serves as a stumbling block; a false God.

My close friend Amanda, twenty-nine, a beauty-shop owner who has previously battled anorexia and bulimia, told me she never weighs herself, *especially* in the gym's locker room. A Reese Witherspoon look-alike with an until-now undiscovered knack for metaphor, Amanda told me the gym scale reminds her of the scale in the deli department of a grocery store, "out there for everyone to see, with a pile of flesh heaped upon it." (Note to self: Substitute tofu for turkey breast on next week's grocery list.) Meat analogies aside, Amanda said her decision to abstain from the scale was the result of a suggestion made by a psychiatrist a decade ago and has served her well—the only time she allows herself to be weighed is at the doctor's office; and even then, she does so standing backward, and on the condition that the number is not uttered aloud. "Psychologically, it's great for me," she said. "Anyway, I use my clothes to gauge my weight."

As does my sister-in-law, Jessica, twenty-six, a Spinning instructor/Harvard MBA student who said she uses the clothes-as-scale technique to avoid becoming reliant on the scale to determine how she feels about herself.

"I get on the scale once a year," Jess said, "and it's something I dread. I think you have this perception in your mind about what you should weigh and when the number comes up, it's depressing, especially for someone like me who works out incessantly. If I lost weight, it might be encouraging and fun, but the downside is actually worse. I guess I just don't want to know the up-and-down, day-to-day, month-to-month of it all."

Jessica is an intelligent young woman who has run the Chicago marathon and hiked the Inca trail, in addition to teaching grueling hour-long Spinning classes to exercise fanatics who demand nothing less than the best. She knows full well that sleek muscle—of which she has plenty—weighs more than fat, even though it takes up less space in clothing. Still, she admitted, "In my deepest thoughts, I think that's just bullshit. I mean, obviously I know it's true, but part of me thinks that saying it is just a way to make myself feel better.

The harsh reality of it is, I don't think I'll ever be 110 pounds. I'm never going to be waify."

Having worked out at two wildly different types of gyms in the past few years—a fancy chain in Chicago as well as her current Ivy League facility—Jessica can attest that the scale rules nationwide. And when women hop on, she finds herself experiencing two reactions. The first, she said, is one of loathing—"Ugh, how can they do that?"—followed quickly by relief that she is not tethered to that slab of steel (unlike the woman in a popular oatmeal commercial who is shown going to work and running errands with a scale chained to her ankle).

"I'm already confused enough by body image," Jessica admitted. "Why add the scale to that confusion? I want to feel good after I work out. If I ran and pushed myself an extra mile or an extra twenty minutes on the Spin bike, I feel good, and part of the reward is that mental release. If I get on the scale, and the number isn't what I want to see, I've just counteracted everything."

What's the Magic Number?

Elizabeth, twenty-four, became a scale junkie while studying abroad. Surrounded by European women who were naturally lean and trim, she was inspired to lose extra weight that, she admitted, needed to come off. Through a routine of intense, two-hour exercise sessions and a strict macrobiotic diet, Liz dropped from more than 200 pounds to 135, her skinniest ever. And even though, upon returning home, she was shocked by some of her friends' reactions, such as those of her male buddies, who admitted to having a difficult time being around her because *now* they were attracted to her (blech), she also found herself loving the stateside locker room's scale. She got plenty of satisfaction from seeing that number—especially when she knew other women were trying to sneak a peek.

"When I weighed that little, I didn't care if people looked," she said. "I kind of wanted them to look. I was proud. I was working really hard—too hard." But because she had spent so much of her life overweight, seeing that number was glorious indeed.

Elizabeth doesn't weigh herself anymore now. She's dropped the restrictive cardio and weight-lifting routines for a more balanced yoga act. The whole idea of numbers, she said, became too restrictive because they began popping up everywhere, not just on the scale. Exercise machines lit up with calories burned, time elapsed, stairs climbed, miles jogged. She was sick of her self-imposed "No eating after 5:00 P.M." rule. Sick of counting every calorie, including each stick of supple gum she folded into her mouth. Sick of weighing herself twice a day. "Numbers," she said, "were my life."

Yoga helped her to become more in tune with her body and its needs. It allowed her to focus on how much energy she needed to have an optimal day, rather than how much energy she'd expended on a machine, which in turn dictated her day. She's now come to realize that her self-image has little to do with other people. It has little to do with the extraordinarily skinny girls who would spring onto the scale, tempting her, in the past, to stare at the scale's readout so that she could compare herself. It has little to do with the European women who sparked her descent into a borderline eating disorder or the American society that fueled it. And it has little to do with numbers. You want to know what it has to do with?

In her short, quirky message on her cell phone, Elizabeth is simply laughing. Laughing so much—genuine giggles so full-bodied that you can literally feel her smile through the phone—that you barely understand what she is saying. But the point is clear: She is happy. Now that's a woman who feels good about herself.

When It's Out of Your Hands

Dara Torres, a model and the winner of numerous Olympic gold medals, didn't have a choice when it came to getting on the scale: Her swimming coach insisted. It started at age eighteen, when she was a freshman at the University of Florida. At first, because weigh-ins were held on Mondays, many of the swimmers, Torres included, would starve themselves on Sundays. When their coach learned about this, instead of getting the girls help (what a silly idea!), he decided to weigh them twice weekly. As a result, the self-imposed starvations doubled. Then the coach started giving surprise weigh-ins and little pop quizzes. How could the girls keep up?

Torres found a way. She became bulimic.

Standing six feet and weighing 155 pounds of mostly muscle, she was still being told to shed pounds so that she would look intimidating on the starting block. During draining training swims, her coach would actually pull her out of the water and feed her chocolates for an energy boost because she was so fatigued from purging in an effort to make weight.

Today, after nine Olympic medals spread out between 1984 and 2000 (she retired for seven years in between), Torres speaks out about her eating disorder and battle with the scale. During her retirement, she weighed herself only once or twice, when she was gearing up to serve as the first female athlete to pose for the *Sports Illustrated* swimsuit issue. Now, at thirty-eight, when speaking to teenagers, she encourages them not to be ashamed about reaching out for help. She's happy that the National Collegiate Athletic Association, the governing body of all collegiate athletics, currently advises coaches to avoid frequent weight and body composition checks. And she never weighs herself.

"There's no reason," Torres said. "I don't want to become consumed. I don't need that stress in my life."

Andrea, twenty-three, wasn't looking for that kind of stress, either, when she joined a gym last year, but she got it when she learned that part of her membership included a mandatory weigh-in with a staff kinesiologist as part of a fitness assessment (which also included a body fat assessment and lab rat–type tasks such as push-ups, sit-ups, and stationary bike riding). Not only was the weigh-in mandatory, but she also had to *pay* an additional $100 for it.

Andrea, an avid Ashtanga yoga practitioner who stands five foot ten and wears a size 8, had not set foot on a scale in more than two years. She was joining the gym for the yoga facilities, not to shed pounds. And yet there she was, her first day, face-to-face with a medical scale as a female staff member urged her to climb on.

"I told her I didn't want to know my weight and she sounded shocked," Andrea recalled. The clash between her yoga philosophy and the more mainstream health club mentality of what women should aspire to was obvious. But, out a cool hundred, Andrea resentfully stepped on the scale.

The kinesiologist's recommendation? Andrea needed to lose 20 pounds. Twenty pounds. Oh, and for further motivation, she also thought it would be a good idea for Andrea to incorporate weight training and forty-five minutes of cardiovascular activity on top of the two hours of regular yoga she practiced. That would probably take her down to somewhere around a size 4. At nearly six feet tall, she'd likely be sapped of the strength to hold a Downward Facing Dog for even fifteen seconds; she could probably manage to slump over in Child's Pose for a while, but that's about it.

Andrea, who typically has a positive self-image and prides herself on her ability to enjoy her curves—contrary to what society dictates—left the weigh-in feeling demeaned and discouraged. She even called her mother and asked (she recalled in a mock crying little girl voice), "Do you think I need to lose 20 pounds?" The scale debacle, Andrea said, was one of the most demoralizing experiences she's had in a very long time.

Sage Is Anything *but* a Number

I had an experience not unlike the aforementioned scale calamity. I had wandered out of my locker room one day and upstairs to my gym's stretching area, where I saw a table set up, staffed by a personal trainer. People clamored all around as he held up a piece of equipment that looked not unlike a Nintendo game piece. On the table, a sign read: "Complimentary body fat testing." Color me intrigued.

I approached the trainer, who explained that all I had to do was grip the two handles, hold the thing straight out in front of me, and the machine would spit out what percentage of my body was composed of lean, calorie-torching muscle and what percentage was horrible, ugly fat. Hmmm. I asked him, "But do you promise it will be *complimentary?*"

"Absolutely," he replied. "No charge."

"No, I understand that," I countered, rather enjoying this grammatical wordplay even though it was, apparently, one-sided. "But I just want to make sure my read-out will be *complimentary.*"

By now a line was starting to form and the trainer's sidelong glance seemed to mutter, "Listen, Crazy Lady, time to shit or get off the pot."

My mind roamed back to the last time I had had my body fat measured. The year was 1998. The place: my hometown of Buffalo Grove. I had just moved back home after graduating from UW–Madison and, what with all the extra income that comes with not having to buy your own tampons or breakfast cereal, I had joined a fancy gym. Part of my initiation fee included a free body fat analysis—this one performed with claw-like metal calipers. I don't know if I was pre-menstrual and bloated or the young man performing my test was some sort of evil sadist or, perhaps (and this is the most likely explanation, I was later assured), he was simply not trained properly. But after pinching the flesh on my upper triceps, abdomen, and thigh, the boy aligned my measurements with some sort of pinwheel-like apparatus and pronounced me . . . morbidly obese.

Suffice it to say, these words were not music to the ears of a recovering anorexic.

Cut to thirty seconds later: There I was, lying on the floor of the aerobics studio, mildly hyperventilating, fat tears rolling down the sides of my face and onto the ground as I sobbed uncontrollably, mumbling something about a pre-gastric-bypass Roseanne Barr. Multiple staff members gazed down at me as if I were a patient on *ER*. A woman assured me the numbers were wrong, that at five foot eleven and 140 pounds, I was *not* morbidly obese.

She helped me up, took me into a private office, gave me a spiel about improper measurement techniques and re-measured my body fat. The new percentage (I honestly don't even remember what it was) apparently assuaged my anxiety enough that I was able to go on to work out for approximately three hours.

Flash back to my current gym. "So, do you want the test?" the trainer asked with exasperation.

You know what I did?

I got off the pot.

2

Booby-Trapped

Hallelujah, My Nipples Have Seen the Light!

It's my first official day on breast patrol and here I am, sitting naked except for two towels—one wrapped around my body, one wrapped turban-style around my hair—and I haven't even worked out or showered. I'm pretending to read a magazine as my nails dry, but really, I'm here to observe, having dedicated the morning to the grand educational pursuit of looking at boobs. Racks. Ta-tas. Hugh Hefner would be so proud.

When you take a few hours to sit down and really study women's breasts (as covertly as possible, mind you—getting caught is about as fun as looking in your rearview mirror on the highway and seeing flashing red-and-blue lights), you see that they exhibit a snowflake-like quality. Not only are no two pairs alike, but every duo is beautiful in its own right. Those that stand at attention signify youth and the promise of a long future, but those that swing low bear the signs of infusing life into children, of fighting gravity for decades and, though losing the battle, of winning the war. From perky to pendulous, barely A to DD, breasts tell a story.

Like so many other women, I consider my upper half my better half. Perhaps that's why I feel so at ease walking to and from the shower or applying my makeup with just a towel wrapped around my waist, but the thought of blow-drying my hair in a baby tee and a thong in public makes me want to vomit. I'm proud of the definition in my arms, which I feel I deserve after logging countless hours in the free-weights room. I feel a certain comfort in the smoothness of my belly. And, yes, I love my breasts. I'm not ashamed to admit it. My name is Leslie and I love my breasts. (Note to all male relatives: Please skip the next paragraph to avoid awkward family reunions.)

Size 36B (though I'm thinking of taking Oprah's advice and getting them measured by a pro), they're perky and ski-sloped, the left one a tad more ample than the right. My areolas are peachy-pink; my nipples an almost exact match to my lips. With a good push-up bra, I can get some respectable cleavage going; au naturel, I can work the Paris Hilton angle. Unlike my plus-sized sisters, I require only one sports bra for when I go jogging and, to the shock of many, during the work week, I can go, shall we say, upper-commando, for days at a time, thanks to the inventor of the shelf bra tank top.

But although I do feel comfortable sashaying topless through the rows of lockers, that doesn't mean I don't compare myself to the endless array of breasts I'm exposed to every day. I admit that I can fluctuate easily between wishing I had Debra Messing's scarcely dipping cleavage to Pamela Anderson's cavernous mountains in a heartbeat, depending on the night/occasion/weather. As the old adage says, we always want what we haven't got on top. Some small-breasted women obtain augmentations (or, if they're on a budget, wedge those chicken cutlet thingies into their bras); more than a handful of large-chested women seek surgical reductions. In fact, breast augmentation and reduction were the second and fifth most popular surgical cosmetic procedures for women in 2005, respectively, according to the American Society for Aesthetic Plastic Surgery.

Whether they're being freed from sweaty sports bras, bobbing around in the air after a shower, or being tucked back into lacy demicups, breasts are unavoidable in the women's locker room; some might say they epitomize it. Like fingerprints, each couple houses its own unique pattern or code. Instead of forever denouncing yours as too big or too small, try to appreciate their distinctiveness: They are natural, beautiful parts of the female body that are all too often ignored by other women for fear the observer will be seen as freaky or (gasp!) a lesbian. In my opinion, it's better to be an open, enlightened pseudo-bisexual than inhibited and uneducated. Look—just don't touch.

Unless you're invited, of course. When personal trainer and all-around spitfire Sonrisa, twenty-nine, decided to acquire breast implants, taking her from "concave" (her words) to a modest, natural-looking 36B (she's extremely lean and muscular and wanted to feel more feminine), the result was a locker room–style free-for-all. The minute one woman asked to feel them and Sonrisa lifted her top, the floodgates opened. She didn't mind; she was very open about the surgery. But *come on,* this was like a large tour of half-naked women going apple-picking; but instead of reaching for apples, they were fondling Sonrisa's new melons.

My friend Randi is actually the one who helped me to become so comfortable with going topless in the locker room. She and I had been in a graduate school course together, the title of which escapes me, though I recall with perfect clarity the ever-present crinkling sounds of her unwrapping her Nutz Over Chocolate Luna Bar. It wasn't until we bumped into each other—literally, and topless to boot—in the locker room of my health club that the seeds of our relationship were planted. We made eye contact: At such an early stage in our relationship, what else could we do? From that glint of recognition sparked a strong friendship.

Maybe it's because Randi, who is thirty-seven, is older than I am (though she still gets carded regularly), and therefore a bit wiser in the body image department, but our weekly chat sessions in the locker room have virtually eroded any sense of discomfort I ever had when looking at other women's breasts. I would say that about 99 percent of our time in the locker room together is spent naked—even when we don't have to be, such as when we're debating whether a model in a JCPenney magazine advertisement is plus-sized or not, or when we're massaging lotion into our dry winter skin. She is so supremely über-confident, not just in her perfect small Bs but in everything she does, that she has changed the way I view my own upper body. Randi loves her boobs and, by association and admiration, I have come to love them too. I can even recognize when she's trying a new birth control pill ("Hey, Rand, lookin' a little perky there today!") and when she's shed a few pounds ("Randelach, what's up with your boobs? Have you lost weight?").

Indeed, when I asked Randi what her favorite part of her body was, she answered, without hesitation, "I dig my boobs." But then, "I also like my arms and shoulders and chest. And I like my ass." As well she should.

Sizing Up "The Competition" (Or, Seeing My Maid of Honor's/Husband's Ex-Girlfriend's Boobs for the First Time)

My husband, Dan, was my best and closest friend for nearly a decade before we married, and throughout that time, he made it fairly clear that he wanted to take our relationship to the next level. Dan is brilliant, hysterically funny, handsome, loyal—everything a girl could want. So I did what any woman in her right mind would do: I ran.

Therefore, it was only a matter of time before he was snatched up by an equally amazing woman: Trish. In fact, I happened to introduce them. That's because Trish was fast becoming one of my closest friends and we were spending a lot of time together. Besides, I was happily dating someone else and it delighted me that these two special individuals were spending time together.

Oh, did I happen to mention that Trish has 36Ds?

I say that not because her breasts had anything to do with Trish's getting together with Dan but because the first time I saw Trish's boobs in their full glory, when I took her to my gym on a day pass, I nearly passed out. My God, were they big! And full. And tan—with no tan lines! Sure, they weren't as perky as mine, but who needs perk when you can strap on a bra and have natural cleavage that tickles your chin? I must admit, when Trish pulled her harness of a sports bra over her head that day in the locker room, my eyes were drawn to her nipples as if by some magnetic force. Blip. Blip. Blip.

If boobs were people, mine were Katie Couric and hers were Marilyn Monroe.

Six months later, Trish and Dan had broken up, my relationship had ended, and I realized that I was ready to start something with Dan. Now, in the past, I've had major jealousy issues when it came to boyfriends' ex-girlfriends. The kind of issues that lead to hyperventilation, crying jags, and one very special knock-down, drag-out fight in a Dairy Queen parking lot. But with Trish and Dan, it was different. I was never jealous, never pictured them in bed together or anything of that sort. If I did, how could I have asked her to be the maid of honor at my wedding?

There were definitely times when I found myself thinking back to that unveiling in the locker room and wondering whether my breasts measured up to the pair he had most recently seen and touched. I never voiced these concerns to either of them, of course, but they existed. Was I too small? Could he settle for wine glasses instead of goblets?

In retrospect, I realize how ridiculous these thoughts were. Dan treats me like an absolute queen; should something horrible happen to my breasts, he would kiss the scars as if they were made of gold. Besides, although Trish and I are both nearly six feet tall (and, admittedly, asked whether we're sisters nearly every time we go out together), our bodies are built too differently to be compared. She is curvy and voluptuous; I'm more athletically shaped. Soon, Dan and I, after ten years of friendship, were engaged to be married and registering at Crate and Barrel . . . for wine glasses.

I learned a valuable lesson here: Although it's difficult not to compare your breasts to those you see in the locker room, try to remember that variety is the spice of life. If we were all 34Bs (or five foot five or red-headed or had the same voice), the world would be a pretty boring place. Men—at least the worthwhile ones—don't actively compare the various body parts of their past and present girlfriends, especially when they're in love. After all, when was the last time you pondered "Oh my God, I'm in love with this man. I think he's the one. But his penis just isn't as thick as my ex's. I think I'll have to pass"? Didn't think so.

A Level Playing Field

My friend and coworker Liz has never lacked for a boyfriend. She's a twenty-nine-year-old petite (we're talking size 5½ shoe), multihued blonde who runs marathons and works out all the time. But what she has always (in her words) lacked are breasts. Her exact bra size is 32A, but she wears a 34A for the self-confidence boost. I've never actually felt Liz up, although she has allowed me to give her padded bra a poke; indeed, my finger pushed through a good inch of material before I hit torso.

Liz is extremely self-deprecating when it comes to her chest, always making jokes at her own expense. But when we sat down for a serious conversation about the topic, her insecurities came pouring out like fizz overflowing from her trademark Diet Mountain Dew.

In the locker room, she said, "I feel like women are thinking, 'Oh my God, she's so small. I feel so bad for her.' It's embarrassing." So embarrassing, in fact, that she always turns around to face the locker when taking off her top. Sometimes she even changes in the bathroom stall. And Liz never, ever walks around without a towel wrapped firmly around her chest. For her, it acts as a shield.

Liz's insecurities about the locker room have carried over into her romantic life. She finds it awkward and uncomfortable when a man reaches to touch her breasts; she's even joked, "Don't bother"—not exactly the most romantic of mood-setters. "Sometimes, I feel like they think they're hooking up with a boy," she said candidly. She doesn't spend money on expensive lingerie, even though she wants to, because she can't fill it out. Liz fears looking silly—like someone she's not.

When asked why she thinks breasts are such a big deal, why she cringes internally when a buxom woman appears next to her in the locker room's mirror to apply her makeup, or when her now fiancé slinks his hand up her back to unhook her bra, Liz said it has to do with what they represent. For her, breasts signify femininity and the qualities that make a woman a sexual being.

But as a card-carrying feminist, Liz recognizes the hypocrisy of her answer. For instance, when she sees a woman at her gym who obviously has breast implants, her reaction ping-pongs between "You go girl, do what you want" and feelings of scorn. On the one hand, she wants to support women in their decisions, even if it means altering their bodies. But then, she also thinks, "If I didn't feel good about myself unless I had fake boobs, I'd be going back on everything I stand for. How could I raise a daughter to feel good about herself if I had those in me?"

Running Around with Circles

Which brings us to Megan, thirty-five, on the opposite end of the breast spectrum. Megan, you could say, is a fairly athletic woman. In 2000, she was the highest-ranked female triathlete in Illinois. She won the 2003 Y-Me Race and the 2003 Race for the Cure. Megan has 13 percent body fat and has been known to run a 5:48 mile . . . for five miles in a row.

One would expect such a lean, mean workout queen to have pecs of steel, but Megan made other arrangements. In 1995, she had her breasts augmented; she ballooned from a 34A to a 34C. That's a little more than half the size of Pamela Anderson's measurement at her fullest, she explained. And though she recognizes she looks a bit out of place at the starting line of her races, she wouldn't have it any other way.

Megan first developed breasts in sixth grade, but she was so active, what with tennis, soccer, cross-country, and swimming, that she burned most of her body fat off, boobs included. And even though she's been an athlete all her life, thin and lean, her mental image has always translated to that of pear-shaped. By the time she was eighteen, she was begging her father for implants to balance out her figure. He didn't buy them for her, so she waited a few years and bought them herself.

Because Megan does a lot of her training outdoors, her activities in the locker room are usually limited to changing clothes and applying her makeup. But she admitted that when she is inside, her chest does offer her a sense of body confidence that she might not otherwise possess. Without her implants, Megan acknowledged she would feel more vulnerable in the locker room.

"There's definitely that underlying current, that need for a competitive edge in the locker room," she acknowledged. "If you weren't happy with yourself, you wouldn't want to be walking around without a towel."

I asked her whether she has ever noticed other women looking at her breasts. Sure, she said with a little laugh. "Especially being an athlete, it's definitely an anomaly to be petite and ripped and have big boobs." At first this answer made me want to loathe Megan just a little bit, probably because I'll never be petite and ripped and have big boobs. But I can't fault her for her honesty (I *can,* however, fault myself for my jealous reaction). Some women, she added, even ask about them, thinking she hit some sort of genetic lottery. But Megan 'fesses up and just outright tells gawkers, "I paid for 'em."

Kasia

Kasia, twenty-eight, a writer who works out regularly but admittedly has a weakness for sub sandwiches and desserts of any kind, has gawked at her fair share of fake boobs in the locker room. But as someone who prides herself on her feminist leanings, she has surprised herself by her bitter reactions. For example, as she was getting ready to work out one day, Kasia, herself a respectable 36C, had just entered the locker room to change when she was confronted by a very slender woman with extremely large, perfectly spherical breasts that exhibited a gravity-defying quality typically seen in mainstream porn. The woman was admiring herself in the mirror, her breasts showcased in a pretty, albeit wholly impractical, sports bra.

"This girl looked as if she belonged on a fashion shoot for *Maxim* magazine rather than in a gym actually working out," Kasia noted. "To draw a silly analogy, it was as if she was out showing off her brand new sports car, not the very nice Toyota Camry that had been in her family all her life and she'd inherited from her mom."

Kasia's immediate response was a mixture of curiosity and repulsion. First, the curiosity: She found herself unable to look away. Not because she felt entranced by the woman's beauty—quite the opposite. (Now, this isn't to say that the woman was not pretty, Kasia pointed out. "She had a beautiful face, blonde hair, and that whole body package so many of us are killing ourselves, both physically and spiritually, to achieve: flat stomach, spindly arms, long slender legs—the works." She also possessed a quality of bizarre artificiality that kept Kasia's green eyes locked in place.)

But any semblance of inquisitiveness soon gave over to feelings of contempt, which Kasia conceded had much to do with her own bodily insecurity. About 30 pounds overweight for much of her adolescence and into her twenties, Kasia, who felt that she carried the extra weight well, still recalls "a generous helping of mean-spirited comments from complete fucking assholes all the way along, including one guy from high school who literally used to moo at me every time I walked past him in the hallway." Even some of her family members harassed her, teaching her to be ashamed of her body rather than to love it.

At twenty-four, Kasia went on a severe diet and dropped 35 pounds in five months. In retrospect, she realizes the method was dangerous, but the outcome was rewarding. People treated her with more respect. Men approached her more often. For the first time in her life, Kasia felt good about her body, and she was inspired to go back into the gym.

So, to see this woman primping in the mirror, her store-bought breasts smooshed together, midriff seemingly effortlessly flat (could've come from thousands of sit-ups; could've come from liposuction), all Kasia could think of was how hard she had to work out while "this girl is at the gym to show off her perfect body and fake tits in a ridiculous outfit she'd likely pop out of if she actually started jogging on the treadmill."

But after that initial rush of anger, Kasia was more annoyed with herself for succumbing, even for a second, to the unattainable body image standards generated by the media and for allowing her insecurities to get the best of her—for allowing another woman's physique to make her feel bad about her own.

So when she was caught staring and the pin-up woman gave her a "you know I'm hot" smirk, Kasia redirected that anger by cutting down the other woman, mentally muttering names such as "stripper" and "bitch" as she changed into her gym clothes. But ultimately, turning the other woman into the enemy didn't help Kasia.

"The fact that she exemplifies the stereotype that has contributed to so much of my pain in the past probably has a lot to do with it. Part of me feels that, by getting fake boobs, she has committed to upholding the artificial beauty standard of our society, to making sure it never changes, to seeing that women like me are never valued as much as women like her."

Kasia has always supported a woman's right to choose what clothes to wear, what birth control to use, what drugs or alcohol to take. You get the picture. So why not plastic surgery, including breast augmentation? What Kasia has realized is that what happened in the locker room that day was deeply rooted in her own body image issues, something she struggles with every day—perhaps more so than she realized.

Liz, Megan, and Kasia might have deviating bra sizes and beliefs, but their need, desire, and response to more oomph in the chest area represents a common cultural belief: When it comes to breasts, bigger is better. And who can blame them? That's what we see every day, whenever we watch television, gaze upon a billboard in Times Square, or read about another gaggle of surgically enhanced *Playboy* bunnies showing up at a Hollywood bash.

Take Two and Call Me in the Morning

I decided to go straight to the source, so to speak, for such surgically enhanced ladies. Robert Rey, MD, a Beverly Hills plastic surgeon, specializes in breast augmentation. Perhaps you've seen him on the E! Entertainment Channel reality show *Dr. 90210,* doing push-ups before surgery and lifting weights while holding his newborn baby. The show chronicles the lives of Los Angeles plastic surgeons and patients as they make their way through boob jobs, liposuction, butt implants, and nose jobs.

According to Dr. Rey, full breasts have been popular since the dawn of time. In the Middle Ages, he explained, breasts were pushed up so high that they practically obstructed a woman's view. They were shoehorned into dresses during Henry VIII's reign, and even farther back, at the time of Jesus, Roman women were stuffing corsets to look a little fuller.

In fact, Dr. Rey continued, women drawn on Indian cave walls were depicted as having full, 500-cc breasts—a small but full D. These are definitely not the kinds of details I learned in fifth-grade history class.

So I get the point: Breasts have forever been in style. And it's not just a West Coast thing: In cities across the United States today, implants are morphing from the oddity to the norm. And why not? In the eyes of Dr. Rey, and of plastic surgeons like him, implants give a woman a competitive edge at a time in history when competition is unparalleled.

"You're kidding yourself if you think looking better does not help yourself in relationships, in jobs, with your self-confidence," Dr. Rey said. "I see it in my office every day. [Women] sit in my chair, don't look in my eye, their voices don't project, their handwriting doesn't project. What's so wrong with putting a little ball with saline water in there and making her feel a little more feminine?" The issue is not one of vanity, he assured me. It's psychology.

Dr. Rey's breast augmentation portion of his practice falls into two main age groups: eighteen to twenty-two and twenty-six to thirty-four. The first group typically comprises girls who had flat chests during their teen years. "They were seen in the high school locker room and the other girls made fun of them. The girls who were fully equipped were the alpha dogs and the flat-chested girls were the omega dogs. It's a hierarchical system. These girls have been thinking about having their breasts done for a long, long time."

The second group—the girls who had larger breasts in high school and who essentially drove the first group of girls to surgery—tend to come in after childbirth, when they are experiencing hormone-driven "shrinkage."

Reporters often challenge Dr. Rey about his tendency to perform larger breast augmentations by asking him, "Would you do this on your daughter?" His somewhat elusive answer: "If a girl is so flat she has no breasts, she gets teased in the locker room, gets teased by her boyfriends, becomes socially withdrawn, would I put a tiny little saline implant in? Yes, absolutely. Just like if her ears protruded out. Would I fix them? Yes."

He continued, "Some girls have outie belly buttons, some girls have a completely flat butt, some girls have vaginal lips five centimeters long. A little tiny tuck below and they feel so much more confident."

Then the final nail in the proverbial coffin: "We cure as much depression as psychiatrists."

I called Marcia Goin, MD, a past president of the American Psychiatric Association, who worked with her late husband, a plastic surgeon, on this very issue. Her take on this bold quote? "Displeasure with one's body is one thing; depression is another. That's different from looking in the mirror and saying, 'Eh, I've got these flat breasts, I don't really like them, I'd like to be more voluptuous.'" In other words, depression is not the same thing as self-consciousness or displeasure with one's body. Nobody's saying a little nip or tuck can't help with the latter. But depression? That often requires help from a doctor who uses his or her pen to take notes or write prescriptions rather than mark up your legs and torso.

Her Cups Runneth Over

But what about the locker room experience for women who feel awkward with *too much* junk in the front? For example, unbeknownst to me, Trish, my fabulously filled-out friend, not only was teased as an early-developing child but is now asked—sometimes by complete strangers—whether her breasts are fake.

Trish admitted she doesn't remember the first time she and I stripped down together, but she's sure she was thinking something to the effect of, "Oh my gosh, I hope she doesn't think I'm gross and have the biggest boobs *ever.*" When in the locker room, she said she almost always attempts to push her chest as far into the locker as possible while taking off her two sports bras. That Trish feels the need to hide what so many others would envy makes me sad. But for her, they're a hassle, a nuisance.

I asked her whether she could recall seeing my boobs for the first time that day in the locker room. She thought about it for a second and said that although she wasn't sure it was the first time she had ever seen them, she remembered being surprised that they didn't touch my torso. "They were completely suspended in midair," she described, as if such a feat were worthy of a Nobel Prize in physics. "I would need some sort of pulley system to achieve that."

That's one of the great things about Trish: She's not afraid to laugh at herself. Sometimes, when it comes to body image issues, mild self-deprecation can help take away the sting of perceived flaws. But naked, Trish is gorgeous. To quote Teri Hatcher in *Seinfeld,* "They're real, and they're spectacular."

When Things Go Awry

What happens when your world goes from spectacular to devastated in the seeming blink of an eye? That's what happened when Susie, a tall, willowy, twenty-nine-year-old blonde in my gym, discovered a lump in her breast. She was on the phone with a girlfriend, laughing so hard she nearly doubled over, and as she put her hand to her chest to catch her breath, she felt it. Upper quadrant of her left breast. The size of an eyeball. Stage 2 cancer.

Because the cancer was self-contained within the tumor, the doctors were able to save Susie's breast by going in under her arm. Radical chemotherapy and radiation caused Susie to lose her hair and, eventually, her energy. But she kept coming to the gym, breathing through the easier yoga positions and gaining stamina from other people's support. For months she wore her wig (she is the woman I spoke of in the introduction); after a while she figured, "Who cares?" and off it came. Having previously battled body-image issues, Susie, now thirty-five and in remission, said, "Going through cancer really makes you wake up and take your focus off those things that are so superficial with your body and moves it onto life or death. It can either destroy you or make you better. That was the gift for me."

For example, she recalled waking up one morning within seven days of starting treatment, taking a shower, and emerging from the tub only to see her hands covered with strands of her long, blonde hair. So she looked up and said, "Susie, you knew this day was going to come. Wipe this shit off your hands, dry your hair, and go to work. You have things to do."

Susie went to work that day, her scalp aching as if she had been wearing an extra-tight ponytail for too long. She then called her brother and asked him to come over later that night and start the process of shaving her head. He agreed, and eight hours later, as he turned the buzzer on, Susie said, "Wait a minute! Do a Mohawk first." So Susie's brother gave her the most loving Mohawk a brother could give. Then he totally buzzed it. That, Susie said, and jumping out of a plane were the two best experiences of her life because they made her feel tough, peaceful, and free.

Susie's breast cancer allowed her to realize that who she is is not her body. "I know the beautiful person I am for real," she explained. "Saying, 'Ugh, I hate my body' is not helping it. You mold your body into the thoughts you have about it." As long as she walks on this earth, Susie intends for the person she projects on the outside to represent the beautiful woman she is on the inside. She cannot, and will not, curse her illness. "Sometimes," she said, "it's what you need to give your ego a swift kick in the butt."

Ironically, the day after buzzing her hair, people at our gym who didn't know about her cancer thought Susie was a model. "You look so strong!" they said. It was a cool, liberating feeling. But then her hair started to get patchy and Susie began to look sick. So she went to a friend's house and shaved her head Kojak-bald.

Meanwhile, cancer was taking a toll on her body image in other ways. She literally lost every piece of hair—eyelashes, pubic, arm, and leg hair. "Like an alien," she described. Not to mention she felt incredibly toxic because of the drugs coursing through her veins.

So she turned to yoga and meditation, visualizing light and crystals and smiley faces flowing through her. She finished her five-year course of Tamoxifen. She took a trip to Las Vegas with her girlfriends and stayed out until 3:00 A.M. every night. The only rough patch came when, while dancing with a man at a club, he started playing with her hair, which was actually a wig. She felt the need to explain, in case something embarrassing happened. It didn't. She's now been cancer-free for more than six years.

She's a Survivor

One of the things I learned while researching this book is that when a breast cancer patient goes in for radiation, she is marked up like a page out of a football playbook. Permanent ink is used to create a bodily graph to show the radiologists where to aim the beams. And as Ronda, a fifty-one-year-old karate teacher and massage therapist also diagnosed with breast cancer, found out, permanent marker ain't easy to get off—even with harsh locker room soap.

So when Ronda changed clothes at the health club in the midst of her radiation, she did so quickly. Even in a sports bra and T-shirt, lines crept out from her sleeves during aerobics class. Though if anyone did ask, she was very open and would simply explain she was in the midst of breast cancer treatment and the lines were guides for the radiologists.

After about a week of treatment, Ronda was lucky enough to get about a half-dozen freckle-sized navy blue tattoos inked across her torso. They served the same purpose as the permanent marker lines, only she still has them, everlasting polka-dot reminders of her battle.

When Ronda was first diagnosed, in 1996, she underwent a right breast lumpectomy. Four years later, her doctors found cancer again, in the same breast. Ronda had already made up her mind that, if the cancer returned, she would have a prophylactic mastectomy on her left side (in other words, have the healthy breast removed along with the cancerous breast). As a karate instructor, balance is important to her, she told me; with just one breast, she would feel truly out of balance. Because she teaches small children and is often in the locker room with them, she had another reason for wanting reconstruction: "I felt it was a very positive body image to present to them: You can go through cancer and survive and maybe even be a new and improved version."

Complications from the radiation prevented Ronda from getting implants; instead, she underwent a bilateral tramflap, a procedure in which a muscle near the belly button is cut, brought up, and reattached to blood vessels near the armpits. Fat is used to form the breasts.

After several self-conscious months, Ronda now has relatively natural-looking breasts, albeit with scars and tattooed, custom-colored nipples. She didn't like any of the stock colors, so she had two blended. Like certain famous celebrities and their lipsticks, she now has a nipple tattoo color named after her. She is happy with her results. In the locker room, she has only noticed other women looking once or twice. It doesn't upset her; rather, she seizes it as an educational opportunity. She also gets about one or two calls a month from other women in her situation. Ronda tells them she came to terms with losing her breasts by realizing it wasn't her arm or her nose or her sight that was being taken away. Her breasts, she felt, had served their function; she had breast-fed her children. In retrospect, she said, "I feel like if my daughter, God forbid, gets breast cancer but has an experience like mine and is able to nurse children and then lose her breast, her life will still be a beautiful, productive life. It will make her a better person."

3

A Waist Is a Terrible Thing to Mind
Eating Disorders Exposed

When I joined my current gym five years ago, it wasn't long before I learned that, along with the perennially fluffed white towels and baby powder-scented spray deodorant, another permanent fixture lingered in our locker room. She was tall and strikingly anorexic looking. Jane's eyes bulged from their sockets and her spandex bicycle shorts actually sagged around her waist and inner thighs. Her dishwater brunette hair had assumed a dry, crimped texture not normally found in nature, parched from what I can only assume (from personal experience and scientific evidence) was a total lack of fat in her diet. I could count Jane's ribs and the spaces between them—visible chasms I had once envied—as if they were keys on a piano. But I hardly ever saw her naked. Unlike nearly every other woman in the locker room, I felt compelled to turn away when Jane undressed.

At that point, I was working out in the mornings and soon learned that Jane, too, exercised early in the day; she just devoted more than triple the amount of time to her sessions that I did, spending an hour on the Stairmaster, then racing through a Spin class, then climbing for another hour on an escalator-type machine. This pattern was repeated, day in and day out, fueled by endless Styrofoam cups of coffee and a will to be thin that had spun beyond her control.

I was in a particularly idealistic frame of mind at that stage of my life and believed I could help women, even if they didn't want to be helped, even if they didn't know they so desperately needed to be saved. I approached one of the physical trainers at the gym—a loud, charismatic guy who seemed to know everyone and who had already introduced himself to me. I explained the situation—that I, someone who had suffered from an eating disorder, was concerned about this woman, who was clearly jogging in place at death's door. Did he think, I asked, it might help if I approached Jane and offered her a shoulder to lean on; an empathetic, formerly anorexic ear that was willing to listen?

His response, God bless him, was brief and blunt.

"I know exactly the woman you're talkin' about," he said in his thick East Coast accent. "You know what she's gonna say if you do that? She's gonna tell you to go fuck yourself."

Oookay.

The trainer went on to explain that Jane had been coming to the gym for nearly a decade. She carried out her triple-hour ritual as regularly as most people shower, brush their teeth, and rush out the door to work. Everyone knew she had a problem, he said—except her.

I craftily tried to appeal to his sense of litigiousness. "What if she has a heart attack on the Stairmaster?" I asked somewhat crossly. "Her family could sue. Surely someone could use that as grounds for the necessity of asking her to get help."

He shook his head. "Americans with Disabilities Act," he shot back. Apparently he'd been through this before. "We can't kick her out."

And so, nearly five years later, Jane continues her anorexic plank walk. She was the first woman I saw in my locker room who suffered from an obvious eating disorder, but she certainly wouldn't be the last.

Observing Jane and recognizing her as a sick woman in need of help was a sentinel event for me. It signified a major step in my ongoing recovery. I no longer envied the wide space between her upper thighs or the dinosaur-like track of spinal vertebrae that jutted out from her back (she makes no attempt to hide her body, within the locker room or outside). And in retrospect, the trainer's response was a major wake-up call. Of course Jane would have told me to go fuck myself. That's the boiled-down essence of an eating disorder: telling the universe—the media, your family, your youth—to stick their idea of perfection and beauty where the sun doesn't shine. Eating disorders are societal challenges. As Mary Pipher, PhD, explains in *Reviving Ophelia: Saving the Selves of Adolescent Girls,* "By her behavior, an anorexic girl tells the world: 'Look, see how thin I am, even thinner than you wanted me to be. You can't make me eat more. I am in control of my fate, even if my fate is starving.'" And this, Jane certainly had accomplished: I have never been able to look at her for more than a moment or two at a time, let alone talk to her about her disorder.

I *have,* however, been able to watch *other* women watch Jane. Their responses range from shock to sadness to disgust. If Jane were out of the frame and one could only view the observer, you might think she was watching a hardcore porn video or rubbernecking a car accident on the side of the highway. You know you shouldn't look—that even just one peek could potentially scar you—but the curiosity is nearly impossible to resist. A naked anorexic woman is a solar eclipse, personified.

I asked Patricia Santucci, MD, executive vice president of the National Association of Anorexia Nervosa and Associated Disorders (ANAD), whether it surprised her that a woman such as Jane, or some of the other extraordinarily thin women in my locker room, do not try to hide their gaunt frames while changing. After all, one of anorexia's textbook characteristics describes sufferers dressing in baggy clothing, layering coats upon sweaters to conceal weight loss. (In fact, that's exactly what I did during my freshman year of college when I topped my favorite baggy moss green J. Crew sweater with the UW tennis sweatshirt I swiped from my first college boyfriend.)

Actually, Dr. Santucci said, she's often been surprised at the number of anorexics who show off their bodies. "They're on the beach, parading up and down in bikinis. It's almost an exhibitionistic quality. It's like, 'Take a look at me.'" A casual flip through a celebrity weekly, filled with paparazzi photos of stick-thin stars in their bathing suits, will confirm that.

Mommy, Why Do You Only Eat Salads?

Much like gay men, who can hone in on other fine young specimens via their "gaydar," many women who have battled eating disorders will tell you they possess a similar sixth sense. It might be the observation of a simple act, such as watching another woman order her lunch ("side salad, balsamic vinegar on the side, squeeze of lemon, please"), or a more obvious, off-the-cuff comment a woman makes about her "huge" size 8 body.

There's a young woman at my gym who seems to follow my workout schedule and, like a man with "gaydar," I was almost positive that she either currently suffered from an eating disorder or had once done so. We exercise with a similar voraciousness and seem to have adopted parallel routines, from our post-work workouts to our shower and makeup rituals. Her stomach is flat and the bottoms of a few of her top ribs—just the bottoms—peek out from beneath her sports bra. I can tell she wears them like a medal of honor, not in an obnoxious way, but with a sense of pride. And I can see that she clings to them as she would to a life preserver. How ironic that the same things that drag us down also seem to keep us afloat.

One day, while undressing, I overheard a conversation in which someone asked this woman to spearhead an intervention with a rather visibly eating-disordered young lady who frequented the locker room. Her reply was indignant; something along the lines of, "It's not my problem. Just because I used to be like that doesn't mean she's my responsibility."

Somehow, I screwed up the courage to approach this woman who, for all intents and purposes, was a stranger. After all, I didn't *really* know anything about her. What if she blew up at me? Told me to, oh, I don't know, *go fuck myself?* To soften the initial impact of my question, I smiled sweetly, introduced myself, and took her to an empty row in the locker room. I asked whether she minded being asked personal questions.

No, not at all, she answered.

Fantastic.

I explained my situation and the research I was conducting and she informed me that she had never had an actual eating disorder. I asked whether she'd mind taking some time to be interviewed anyway—even anonymously. Unfortunately, she declined. As she said, she'd never had an eating disorder.

Yet without further provocation, over the next few minutes, she told me that she had once been downing up to eight laxatives a day, was currently on a pretzel-based diet, considered herself an exercise bulimic (somebody who compulsively over-exercises in an attempt to compensate for calories consumed), could not make herself throw up but wished she could and had recently been asked by her young son, "Mommy, why do you only eat salads?"

Eating Disorders by the Numbers

Mommy is far from alone. Ours is a culture so terrified of fat that, in a recent study conducted by a consortium of genetic health services providers, 11 percent of Americans said they would abort a fetus if genetic testing showed it would grow to be an obese person. More than eight million women suffer from eating disorders, according to the National Association of Anorexia Nervosa and Associated Disorders, and countless more practice various eating-disturbed behaviors. Take, for instance, one of the models on a popular television show who, at five foot ten and 130 pounds, commented that her intermittent vomiting after meals did not render her bulimic. Equally common are girls and women who skip meals or are overly obsessed with food and body image in general. Such behaviors have been shown to preface full-blown eating disorders, 86 percent of which manifest themselves before the age of twenty. Eating disorders are the third most frequent chronic illness among adolescent females and, at 6 percent, carry the highest fatality rate of all psychiatric illnesses.

Just think about that for a second: *The highest fatality rate of all psychiatric illnesses.*

That so many eating disordered women, obvious or not, slip through or at times strut about my well-kept locker room is a testament to the prevalence of anorexia, bulimia, and other eating disorders in middle- and upper-class women. Less economically endowed individuals often cannot afford, financially or emotionally, to refuse food; it would be a futile way to cope with strife. And so, ironically, those who are better off starve themselves until they have collarbones that could slice the finest of cheeses, but refuse the cheese as if it were poison.

Indeed, membership to my gym isn't cheap at about $120 a month. Members are women and men who, more likely than not, were raised in financially well-off families; now they have the disposable income to purchase a vast array of products and services conducive to a preoccupation with weight, such as health club memberships, fashion magazines, diet foods, and plastic surgery. Eating disorders' prevalence amongst women of the upper socioeconomic strata—the women in my locker room—is a prime example of the adage "starving in the midst of plenty." As author of *The Body Project* Joan Jacobs Brumberg, PhD, has put it, the epidemic is "consistently restrained by age and gender but promoted by social mobility."

For instance, my friend Sara, a petite, voluptuous twenty-nine-year-old who has struggled with anorexia and bulimia on and off for more than a decade, is a high-powered businesswoman. And the lady who reminded me so much of myself, the one who eats nothing but salads? She's an architect. Successful, intelligent women, controlled by the mirror.

Just Stick Your Finger
Down Your Throat and to the Left

Darlene's friend Jenny taught her how to make herself throw up in the locker room after ballet class one day when she was nineteen. A sophomore at an all-girls college, Darlene envied her senior friend's perfect body and seeming ability to eat whatever she wanted. One day she asked. Jenny simply laughed and said, "I can show you how you can eat all you want and not gain any weight."

Locked in a stall together, Jenny taught Darlene how to purge. "She said, 'Just stick your finger down your throat and to the left.'" And much to Darlene's surprise, "Instead of thinking it was the grossest thing ever, I remember feeling powerful. We had Thanksgiving dinner and then went and threw it up."

That was twenty-two years ago. Now married with a six-year-old daughter conceived through in-vitro fertilization (the damage done by decades of on-and-off starving and vomiting made natural conception too difficult), Darlene still has a difficult time entering the locker room. After an aerobics class, she'll hang back for an extra ten minutes for other women to clear out, not because she's uncomfortable about changing clothes but because the typical locker room banter tends to veer away from encouraging remarks—such as "Oh, how are your kids doing?"—and toward the more downbeat "What did you eat today?" and "I'll never get that ice cream sundae off my butt."

In retrospect, Darlene said, although that ballet class twenty-two years ago was supposed to be a healthy activity, it was probably one of the worst days of her life. She wishes she could "just black it out."

This comment illuminates the critical need to know where you stand, emotionally, when you enter the locker room. It's kind of like going out drinking with your girlfriends: You have to have some sort of plan—an idea of what you want to wear, whether or not you want to hook up, and whether you want your friends to reel you in if you start climbing on the bar and grinding against Lord knows who. Otherwise, your beer goggles might lead you home to shack up with a total stranger—not a smart move in itself—and the result could be far worse than a raging hangover and a humiliating stumble of shame back to your apartment. On the other hand, you could stay in control, toss back a few Effen cherry vodka and 7-Ups, flirt like a madwoman, then hit the local all-night diner to dish with your friends.

As in the bars, the environment of the locker room can offer a mood-boosting or mind-busting experience, depending on your self-image and where you fall on the spectrum of eating disorders. If you can accept various body sizes and shapes, as well as your own, the locker room can be a healthy place, Dr. Santucci said. But for women carrying matching sets of emotional baggage, it can become a testing ground of sorts. "If she has the perspective that she must be a

size six and you should be able to see her pelvic bones stick-
ing out, then the locker room becomes a dangerous place in
some ways." Unfortunately, Darlene fell into the latter category. But she's making the long climb out.

The Locker Room Bond

I had seen Sara, the businesswoman I spoke of earlier, many
times before, dressed in (or should I say, stripping out of)
sassy outfits of tailored blazers, expensive jeans, camisoles,
pearls, and high heels. Always wheeling and dealing on the
phone or chatting with other locker room regulars, Sara
seemed impressive and easily approachable.

One day while applying our makeup, I noticed her perfume: lime, sugar—a mojito for the pulse points. I had to ask.
She shared a spritz, and, with that cloud of Burberry Brit, our
friendship blossomed.

The next time we worked out, we grabbed side-by-side
elliptical machines; as we sweated, we spilled our deepest
secrets like red wine on a white chenille throw. For me, this
was nothing new; but Sara punctuated every breathless sentence with "I can't believe I'm telling you this" and "My husband doesn't even know this!" (They were going through a
divorce at the time.) We spoke mostly of our past eating disorders and current struggles with body image. We compared
notes and soon found that we were both Jewish and that our
fathers were entrepreneurs in the food industry. We both
sought refuge in running. And we had both hit our rebel-
lious periods much later in life than most people.

I later asked Sara why she felt she could open up so
quickly to me and tell me things, say, about her bulimia that

she had never revealed to her husband. She, too, spoke of the elusive bond of the locker room.

"You see the same people every day, over and over again, for years in that locker room," she said. "You think, 'I see these people more than my own families.' They become your friends . . . especially as they are all women."

Sure, that might account for the ease with which friendships form, but what about the intimacy that had been injected into ours?

"There's something about that environment," she said. "People who are at the gym as much as I am, I don't think it's just for health reasons. I think maybe we share some kind of common background." So perhaps she was drawn to me because she saw in me something she knew existed in her. A shared sisterhood; someone who could understand.

Eating on the Run

Two days before Christmas, Katherine, twenty-nine, was taking part in a circuit training session—one of those classes where you dash from machine to machine, trade free weights for a run on the treadmill, stomach crunches for lat pull-downs. She was up for a ten-minute segment on the Spinning bicycle, but had forgotten the foot clips that help ensure your feet stay attached to the pedals as they whirl around at breakneck speed. Still, the pedals did have cages, which work in a similar fashion, only not as securely.

Somehow in the middle of her workout, as Katherine followed the instructions to rise up from her seat and cycle quickly while standing, the right pedal flipped over—with the top half of her right foot caught in the cage. Screeching to an awkward, excruciating halt, she tumbled off the bike, grasping for the handles and crying out for help. Once the girl next to her had helped untangle her from the bike, Katherine's ankle immediately and angrily swelled up. She was given some paperwork to complete (no doubt filled with health club legalese) and, too embarrassed to ask for help, she hobbled out of class.

Her doctor fitted her with an air cast and crutches for what was diagnosed as a severely bruised ankle bone and two or three torn ligaments.

A few days later, Katherine was walking on the treadmill. Soon she was on the recumbent bike.

"Everybody thought I was crazy," she admitted. But the lack of exercise was driving her stir-crazy and she just needed to *move*. I understood how she felt. Most women who have had eating disorders would know how she felt.

But Katherine does not have a conventional eating disorder. She has, in her words, "a bingeing thing." Not in a sit-on-the-bedroom-floor-lock-the-door-and-surround-yourself-with-cerealmilkchipsicecreamandfishsticks-PBS-afterschool-special-kind-of-way. More like sneaking treats behind closed doors and then punishing herself at the gym for four hours. Or going shopping with her boyfriend, buying a cookie, hiding it in her pocket, and then secretly eating it in the store's bathroom. And then she works out for a long time. "Emotional eating," she called it.

This sounded so blatantly like exercise bulimia to me that I couldn't help but blurt out my layperson's diagnosis. At first she was silent. Then she told me she had never heard of that phrase but that she had never been anorexic or bulimic. Still, food and exercise *have* always been on her mind. And then, in perhaps the most sadly poetic turn of phrase I've yet to hear, she said, "I don't know whether that's an eating disorder or just part of being a woman."

After about four months of pain—both physical, from the injury, and emotional, from not being able to work out with the passion with which she would have liked (but working out nonetheless)—Katherine had surgery to repair her ankle. She simply could not stand being away from her runs, her volleyball league, her near-daily workouts.

Please, don't get me wrong. I'm not trying to lambaste her—not in the least. I, too, am a workout junkie, and I'm not in the habit of calling kettles black when I am the pot. Like Katherine, I understand the compelling and constant need to feel sweat spring from my pores and my heart pump fast and strong. And, as Katherine noted, if I were injured, I would probably feel the need to wear the air cast to justify to others why I was walking and not running on the treadmill.

Thankfully, the ankle surgery was a success, but Katherine had to stay off of her right foot for another four weeks. The process, she said, "nearly killed me."

Living Life Large . . . and Loving It

In addition to the brave women sharing their stories above, I knew there was one famous story I had to include: that of Kate Dillon. Perhaps you recall seeing Dillon in *People*'s "50 Most Beautiful People" issue alongside Julia Roberts and Charlize Theron in 2000, or in a steamy Gucci ad, or on the cover of *Mode Magazine*. At five foot eleven and ranging between 160 and 170 pounds, Dillon is one of the most successful plus-sized models on the planet—never mind the fact that, at a size 14, she wears the same size as the average American woman.

But Dillon didn't always feel this comfortable with her body. In 1984, when ten-year-old Dillon moved with her family from the East Coast to Southern California, dieting became a new coping mechanism as her body packed on the pounds in preparation for what was about to become a major growth spurt. But by the seventh grade, she had shot up six inches and lost 30 pounds; when she was seventeen, she was "discovered," placing third in *Elite*'s "Look of the Year" contest (prize: a $75,000 contract), and was soon in Paris doing runway and print modeling.

Unfortunately, Dillon found herself thrust into a bizarre world of delusion where even a size 4 can be too big. "I remember one season, this *Harper's Bazaar* editor saying, 'You look so great,'" Dillon recalled, "and I remember thinking, 'I haven't eaten in ten days.' I began to question my behavior and my belief system. We were working very hard to create an illusion that didn't exist. As someone who had had an eating disorder since she was twelve years old . . . drinking coffee, smoking tons and tons of cigarettes, going to weigh myself in the middle of the night. I thought, 'Here I am, I'm a part of this illusion machine.'"

Dillon decided she did not want to be part of that machine—this same sick structure that fuels everyday women in the locker room to compare themselves to the very magazine spreads Dillon was starring in as a teenager. She hired a nutritionist, got out of the modeling industry, and returned home to soul search and "come to terms with this new body" that had put on upward of 50 pounds.

"I had a spiritual awakening," Dillon said. "I began to feel liberated from deep within." No longer did she wish to be subjected to other people's ideals of beauty—she made a conscious decision, she said, to "not be embattled," to believe that not only was she going to accept herself, "but I am going to change the way I perceive my body and decide that being five foot eleven and 170 pounds is fine and having cellulite is fine and having saggy boobs is fine."

Apparently a good part of society agrees, because when Dillon moved back to New York at twenty-two and a friend suggested plus-sized modeling, she was signed immediately. And now she's making bank.

At her current size, Dillon is an internationally renowned model and she has the world at her feet. She hikes, she does yoga, she's healthy. She can eat ice cream if she so chooses, the real kind. She has a boyfriend. She's hot. Think about it: She's comfortable in her own skin, and that makes her sexier than a strut down a Paris runway ever made her.

"I about died," she admitted, of being told by her agent that she had been named to the list of all lists, *People* magazine's "50 Most Beautiful People"—at her higher weight, not her "skinny-model weight." Not because she didn't consider herself beautiful, and not because she doesn't still have days when she wishes she were a size 2, but because of the implication. "There I was with Julia Roberts," she proudly remarked. "It made such a neat statement about beauty and inclusiveness and the world. We were always the ugly stepsisters and suddenly we were *there*."

But despite her eventual conquering of her eating disorder and praise and support from women—and men—worldwide, Dillon still covers up in the locker room. She theorized that perhaps she does so because of her locale: She lives in Texas, where social values tend toward the conservative side. But in her own words, "In the locker room, I'm more conscious that maybe somebody else doesn't want to see me naked."

At first, my jaw dropped when she told me this—it sounded as if Dillon, the woman who moments earlier had proclaimed that, upon entering the plus-sized modeling world, she was "going to turn this business on its head, because I knew you don't have to be skinny to be awesome"— sometimes had moments of self-doubt. But upon further clarification, she explained it had nothing to do with her weight; rather, it was a reaction to society's general attitude toward nudity. "It's not because I have anything to hide," she said. "I'm just aware of other peoples' prudishness. People are weird about nudity. They don't want to look at another woman's body." But should Dillon's towel fall, she will simply pick it back up, sling it over her shoulder, and strut her stuff to the showers.

Dillon likes to emphasize to other women of all ages and sizes that, when deciding how you want to live your life, you should make a conscious choice to find out who you are and, more importantly, celebrate it. What are your strengths? What are you really good at? Cultivate those skills. Do some self-reflection, Dillon urged. That way, you can move on from figuring out what makes you sweat to finding out what makes you glow.

4

I Scream, You Scream, We All Scream for . . . a $50 Bikini Wax?

Locker Room Beauty Rituals

Y ou never forget your first time.

For me, it started out just as I had imagined it. I was nervous, yes, but excited, too. It seemed to be my true entry into womanhood. I had missed my opportunity in college— you know, the "experimental years"—but I had always wanted to try it, so I was grateful that this was going to be with someone more experienced. She was tall, blonde, and slender, and graciously gave me a few moments of privacy to disrobe. "Breathe deeply, Leslie," I thought to myself. "This is what you wanted. It's going to feel so good after the shock wears off. You'll feel so sexual, like such a real woman."

I lay down on her clean white sheets, the dimmed lights and soft music soothing my nerves. And then, a knock at the door.

"May I come in?"

"Umm, y-yes."

At first, there was a bit of fumbling. I shivered from being cold and, I suppose, my nerves, so she covered my top half with a soft towel. There, that was better. Almost instinctively, I pulled my legs up so my knees were bent, my feet just a few inches from my rear. My eyes were closed so it surprised me at first to feel a pair of hands on my upper thighs.

"Okay, now just open your legs a bit for me . . . "

Ohmygod, was this really happening?

"Now, you're going to feel something warm inside your right leg."

There was no turning back now. It was really happening. Oh shit, what would my father think? This was the same guy who always told me to put an aspirin between my knees on a first date and never let it fall.

"Leslie, I need you to pull your right thigh back by your ear and let your left knee fall down to the side. And take a deep breath."

And then, my life flashed before my eyes. Holding my baby brother for the first time. Toddlers laughing on swing sets. Finger-painting at my grandparents' house. Barbie dolls. Halloween. Horseback riding with my father. My Bat Mitzvah. My first kiss. Drunken college nights starting with Jello shots and ending with cheese fries. The wedding I hadn't had yet. And a bright light at the end of the tunnel.

This was my Brazilian bikini wax and I had asked for it. Paid for it, actually. It took place in a private massage room in my locker room. When it was over, my cha-cha looked as if it belonged in *Playboy*. Yowza. It was like some sort of vaginal topiary. For a moment, the pain was replaced by an undeniable urge to touch the sculptural wonder, much like a child at the museum yearning to pet the magnificent dinosaur behind the ropes, even though she knows the risk of being kicked out. But before I could do anything, a request from the aesthetician erased the dazed smile from my face.

"Pull both of your legs back like a baby so I can wipe the extra wax off and powder you." I am not lying, these were her exact words. So much for feeling like a woman.

It is at moments like these that I wonder, "Why the hell am I doing this?"

Can We Makeup?

The answer, of course, is beauty. Whatever we do in the gym, from lifting weights to swimming laps to climbing endless stairs, sure, we can say we're doing it for our health. And maybe we are . . . in part. We want to stave off heart disease, keep our bones strong so we don't age into hunched-over little old ladies, keep cancers of all kinds at bay. But whether we like to admit it or not, vanity is a key element in our exercise routine. We don't strive for toned thighs and a tight ass with just a reduction in arterial plaque in mind. It's beauty, baby. Admit it. And after our sweaty session is blessedly over, our pursuit of pretty perfection continues in the locker room.

Lotions and potions, pots of crème applied sparingly in some places, liberally in others. Brown sugar or Dead Sea salt scrubs for unearthing smooth skin; alpha hydroxy acids to smudge away wrinkles. Women's makeup bags spill onto the locker room's counters, shadows and liners and lipsticks rolling every which way, like children scattering at recess. Flatirons and curlers, fancy Mason Pearson brushes and cheap plastic combs soaking in aqua-tinted, antiseptic-filled glass jars. Enough hair product to make Pamela Anderson's trademark coif seem downright uninspired. Self-tanning spray and bronzer. And fragrances mingle until you can't tell a floral oriental from a vanilla musk from a fruity body refresher.

And, of course, there are the noises that accompany these beauty rituals: the sharp, stomach-turning clipping of some-one else's nails followed by the back-and-forth grating of fil-ing. The snapping sound of compacts closing. Club-provided aerosol hairspray cans hissing away while lotion bottles squirt out sounds vaguely reminiscent of sex or some less sa-vory bodily function. Makeup bags unzipping and zipping back up, their teeth gobbling the cosmetics as voraciously as the owner herself. Lips emitting that trademark gooey air kiss sound as they pucker and smudge the gloss just so. Perfume bottles spritzing. From behind the closed aesthetician's door, you might hear the dreamy "mmmm" of a massage or the sti-fled scream of a waxing. And drowning out everything is the poor girl who has to bear the unfortunate beauty cross of aiming not one but two hairdryers at her head to leach the water from her extra-thick locks.

Sure, some of us are wash-and-go natural nymphs, ready to run with a quick shampoo and spray of mountain fresh de-odorant, courtesy of the gym. (So *that's* where my dues go.) And yes, many times, that person is me, especially during those unbearable Chicago summer nights when it's too hot for a blow-dryer, too sticky for a bra, and I simply cannot bear the thought of getting back into my business casual dress and heels. On those days, I shower, shave, stick some toilet paper on the nickel-sized divot of skin I've inevitably gouged from my shin with the locker room's razors, and throw on what will essentially become my pajamas for the night: a baby-soft shirt with some slogan that only I and maybe three other people on Earth think is funny—for example, a Hungry Hippo from the 1980s standing up, shrugging his shoulders, and explain-ing, "I just wasn't that hungry-hungry" (don't think the irony of my wearing this is lost on me); a pair of Gap cotton pajama shorts; and flip-flops.

But more often, you'll find me engaging in at least a few beauty practices after my workout. I've got my shower routine down pat, including my special hair products for chemically treated blondes (you didn't think this nice Jewish girl's highlights were from the *sun,* did you?); Lever 2000 soap, because I sweat more than Michael Jordan but adore smelling super shower fresh; and Jergens lotion containing some self-tanner, which I alternate with Bath & Body Works body cream—Cucumber Watermelon in the warm months, Sweet Pea otherwise.

Because I tend to work out in the evenings, makeup isn't an issue unless I'm going out. So I just slick on some Rosebud Lip Salve, work out the tangles from my fine (as in thin, not awesome) hair, and I'm on my way.

On the other hand, my friend Eden, who is thirty, belongs to one of the most exclusive gyms in town and chooses to wake up early and work out in the morning. While I'm hitting the snooze alarm, she's emerging fresh-faced from her locker room's shower. Her routine now seems incredibly ironic because when we were college roommates she would slam her snooze button over and over, as if she were playing the Whack-a-Mole game at Chuck E. Cheese.

Eden has her shower routine down to an exact science. We're talking organic chemistry. It begins when she hangs her sweaty clothes on hooks in her locker to air out; she then grabs three fluffy towels—one to wrap around her ample chest, one around her very tiny waist, and one to drape around her neck. Slipping into her flip-flops, Eden grabs her hot pink shower tote decorated with black bustiers and filled with coconut-scented Paul Mitchell products, body wash, a pouf, and other assorted items. And off to the showers she goes, stopping only for a razor on the way.

She foams her bod up with a grapefruit-and-pear body wash and massages in her favorite shampoo. When she's thoroughly fruity and cleansed, she rinses from head to toe. Next, ignoring the advice of hair stylists everywhere, she uses a *brush* to untangle her wet, curly red hair. Then comes some acne soap for her back and Paul Mitchell finishing rinse. While that sinks in, she uses a footstool to shave her legs with women's shave gel. Pits, too. After a final rinse comes the entertaining part; this has been with Eden for years. She wrings out her hair as if it were a towel, then whips it up and down, up and down, and from side to side; she looks like a spastic, naked, redheaded punk rocker. She believes this routine helps pull extra water to the ends of her hair, which she then wrings out again. It's a miracle she has not given herself a concussion by doing this in the confines of her shower stall.

After drying off, her hair wound in a turban, Eden heads straight to the mirror to "lube up" with Lubriderm SPF 15 on her arms, legs, face. Next, straightening crème in her curls helps avoid frizz. Then it's back to the lockers to dress and apply makeup.

A self-described "makeup snob," Eden has a face that lives the good life, courtesy of her fabulous older sister, who's employed by Barneys. Perched at the locker room's vanity, Eden uses only the best: Chantecaille foundation, Nars blush, Vincent Longo bronzer (I swear, I haven't name-dropped this much since my clubbing days of the early 2000s), Sue Devitt eyeliner and mascara, and Fresh lip gloss.

Susie, the woman who survived breast cancer, also has an elaborate locker room beauty routine filled with rather pricey products, but the reasoning behind her rituals is rooted in more than aesthetics. After her cancer experience, Susie made some major life changes that included eliminating animal byproducts and mineral oils from her beauty supplies. She probably watches as women (myself included) pump lotion out of the giant tubs provided by the club and pictures us smearing mayonnaise on our limbs and torsos.

Susie's beauty routine starts with a stint in the dry sauna about four times a week, then a trip to the showers with an assortment of organic, holistic products, including a low-preservative soap, a loofah, a shampoo that looks like something you might scrape off your boots after a camping trip and is made of sea minerals (it takes me a few seconds before I realize she's not saying "semen," but with earth-mother Susie, one never knows), and a fruit-based conditioner from Whole Foods. I get the feeling that if I were stranded on a desert island, I could survive by eating Susie's shower products alone. Well, that and my mayonnaise lotion.

But it's the skin-care routine that sets Susie above and beyond all other women. As a consultant for a line called Arbonne, she has a vested interest in their skin-care line that quite possibly has more steps than a certain famous alcohol and drug addiction program. It starts with a spray of facial toner, then a layer of facial serum, which is like an eye gel but for the whole face. Next comes the body serum, body lotion, and eye cream. While these various organic potions are soaking in, Susie heads over to her locker to get dressed halfway. Then, it's back to the vanity, where she smoothes on the daily lift product and blow-dries her long, blonde hair. Interestingly, Susie's hair was very thin and straight before she started chemotherapy, but after falling out, it grew back in luscious, thick Shirley Temple ringlets. Now the curls have relaxed into more of a loose wave, but still, isn't it bizarre how the body works?

Next comes a day cream with SPF 8, some foundation (I'm not sure why, because her complexion is gorgeous), and a little lip liner. "That's it," she joked. "Total ritual."

I asked Susie whether strangers ever say anything to her about the multiple facial and body tonics she has lined up on the locker room counter like her own little personal war on aging. She said sometimes she does catch a woman peeking over, as if she were cheating on a test and trying to see just what the answer is. "You just know when somebody's watching and is like, 'What the hell is she doing?'" Regardless, Susie believes that women are mindful of what products and beauty rituals other women are using and partaking in, just as we're interested in what the butt or belly of the girl at the locker next to ours looks like. Essentially, it's a grading game.

"If they think the other person's beautiful, maybe they'll pay more attention." Which rings true for me: I'll contort my neck to peek into a pretty girl's makeup bag to see what kind of bronzer she just used, just as I'll try to catch a glimpse of her skirt size when she folds it up and places it in the gym bag. Sure, it's embarrassing, but I'll cop to it. However, I've also been known to play a made-up drinking game with my friend Amanda in which we guess the calorie and fat content of random items in our kitchens, too, so that doesn't mean it's necessarily the healthiest thing to do.

If beauty in the locker room were, indeed, a grading game, then sixty-eight-year-old health club owner Hazel gets an A. She doesn't spend much time in the locker room itself, for her business is behind the scenes and on the floor of the gym. But when she does sweep through the entrance, her presence is often cause for excitement. A beauty pageant winner growing up—at sixteen she was even voted "Most Head Turningest Girl" of her high school—Hazel still has what it takes (she was fifty-one when she won her last beauty contest). Hazel always wears perfectly applied lipstick, a lesson instilled by her mother, and when she passes through the locker room she is often stopped by other women asking for makeup tips and such.

"People know I've been in this business for a long time and I give them answers," she explained with a mix of pride and modesty. "I've been asked about my perfume or to tell them the product I'm using." And she does so with pleasure.

Maybe you recognize yourself in Eden and Susie with their elaborate beauty routines and pricey products. Or in Hazel, in her willingness to share beauty tips with fellow gym-goers. Or maybe you identify more with the young mother who, juggling a crying kid on her hip and a bulging gym bag slung over her shoulder, dashes out the door in her flip-flops, wet hair stuck to naked cheek. Perhaps you fall somewhere in the middle, like Carissa, thirty-one, who admitted that a part of her "feels it would be really cool to be one of those low-maintenance girls who can just rub a bit of gel into her hair—*whisk, whisk*—and be on her way." But Carissa still uses a curling iron every morning, so her days of being a "whisk, whisk" girl are far in the future. "I feel ashamed confessing I use it," she said. "It's like admitting I still live in Laura Ingalls Wilder land."

Talkin' 'bout Evolution

It's comes as no surprise that we women are constantly physically fine-tuning ourselves, be it eyebrow or bikini waxing, exfoliating facials, French manicures, or the finest creams and lotions that money can buy. All in the pursuit of what? Attracting a mate? Looking prettier than the next woman? Feeling better about ourselves?

Helen Fisher, PhD, an anthropologist at Rutgers University and author of *Why We Love: The Nature and Chemistry of Romantic Love,* is so deeply embroiled in answering these kinds of questions that she has performed scientific experiments that involve scanning the brains of couples who are madly in love. In men, she has found, certain parts of the brain light up like a Christmas tree when pictures of their sweethearts are flashed before them.

The bottom line, she said, is that men are real lookers—and she doesn't mean head-turners. Men like to watch, and they've been looking at women for millions of years, mainly for signs of youth and fertility.

Here's where the beauty rituals come in. Those golden highlights you pay $150 for every two months? You may not consciously know it, but blonde hair symbolizes youth, Fisher said—which, in turn, the core male mind sees as an opportunity to spread his seed and produce. (And you thought that the saying "Blondes have more fun" just meant getting more appletinis bought for you.) And that eyeliner and mascara you so deftly apply as you sit at the vanity? What we (my makeup bag contains no fewer than ten eggplant, black, brown, and sage eyeliners) are subconsciously doing is trying to make our eyes look bigger and rounder, like a baby's. I know this sounds bizarre, but think about it: As Dr. Fisher explained, children have very large eyes in relation to their skulls. Think Barbie, think Kewpie doll. By trying to mimic that appearance (Hollywood starlets and porn stars alike are guilty), women are emitting a baby-like, youthful signal associated with fertility. And we've been doing it for three thousand years.

Then there's lipstick, one of my favorites. We slick it on, all those glossy reds, pinks, and peaches. Sometimes we draw slightly outside our natural lip line to make them appear more plump, or have any number of chemical or "natural" fillers injected into them to puff them up. Companies put cinnamon or other irritants in their glosses to make our kissers swell. We idolize Angelina Jolie's bee-stung chopper toppers. Ever wonder why? As Dr. Fisher explained, when we were primates, sauntering from club to bar on all fours, our genitals were easily seen by the opposite sex. We all had Brazilian bikini waxes! But once we went bipedal, women's fancy bits got tucked away, never to be seen again.

The way anthropologists see it, by coloring and enhancing the lips on our face, we are actually reminding men of the lips that await down below. In fact, I've even heard that if a woman whips out her lipstick at dinner while on a date and brazenly applies it in front on him, it's an indication of naughty things to come . . . catch my drift?

"Women spend their lives trying to look good for men," Dr. Fisher said, describing us as, essentially, walking billboards. And we're not just advertising for the fellas but for "other women, for our bosses, for friends. Some people are advertising that they're intellectual or jocks or good mothers or sexy and available for an affair." And it's not just makeup: Clothing, hair, perfume all send incredibly powerful messages about our social status, our level of wealth, our availability, and our potential as a mate. Even something as simple as the blue jeans we pull on after a workout, Dr. Fisher said, make a statement, become an advertisement for how much money we have.

The process of choosing the jeans of the moment over Wranglers, Chanel over Wet 'n' Wild, is likely not conscious (in terms of scoring a partner); Dr. Fisher believes that "if you ask a woman why she puts on makeup, she'll say because she wants to look better. [However], for millions of years, those women who coifed themselves to look better won more mating opportunities, had better husbands, and passed on their own genes associated with being motivated to look good." Just as a male peacock fans out his tail feathers, all kinds of creatures go to great lengths to impress the opposite sex, and even the same sex. It's survival of the hottest—at its most literal sense in the health club locker room.

On Hair

I. Sadowaxokistic

Elisabeth Flynn, thirty-four, has been an aesthetician for twelve years, first working for a plastic surgeon in Nashville, and now in the locker room of my gym. She's that tall, thin blonde who gave me my first Brazilian experience. So it was with a bizarre mix of embarrassment and journalistic conviction that I contacted her to discuss why it is, she thinks, women go about having their pubic hair ripped from the follicles with hot wax.

Though Flynn performs facials, glycolic peels, and eyebrow and lip waxes in our locker room's salon, she revealed that bikini waxes are far and away the most popular service—especially those of the landing-strip variety. She attributed

their popularity to today's shrinking bathing suits and underwear. No one wants to see tufts of hair peeking out from behind an itsy-bitsy teeny-weeny yellow polka-dot bikini.

Also, Flynn said, customers like the clean, hygienic feeling
that accompanies a fresh waxing. And, I must admit, there's a
certain sensuality that accompanies the experience. After my
first time, even just pulling on my jeans felt good . . . and I
hadn't even started walking yet! Once I hit the streets, it was
like my little secret. Every time I passed someone, I thought,
"Hey, Baby. Guess what I just did." Although the first time I
went *totally* bare, I remember going to use the locker room's
bathroom, pulling down my gym shorts, and momentarily
frightening myself with what appeared to be a three-year-
old's vagina. "Pedophile!" I chastised myself inside.

Flynn admitted the first-time interaction can be fun, if the
client is cracking jokes or has a sense of humor about the experience. And hopefully she has one, because when you're
being placed in Cirque du Soleil contortions by a stranger
and you ain't wearing nothing but a T-shirt, a sense of humor
is your best defense. That and a glass of wine, which apparently some clients slam back before the moment of truth. Aspirin can help, too, she said. Valium, anybody?

The number one reason women cite for having the procedure is to please or surprise their significant others, Flynn
said. Oh, the things we do. But after the first time, "they like
the clean feel, so that brings them back." Some women might
request a shape, such as a heart for Valentine's Day (do they
style menorahs for Hanukkah?) or even their man's first initial. I'm guessing "T" for Tim is easier than "B" for Brian. One
of Flynn's colleagues even has a lady who wanted to wear a
specific pair of white pants to a special event, but underwear

was out of the question; so instead, out came the wax. A total wax at my gym costs $45 plus a 20 percent tip, and those pants probably cost at least $100, so the woman had better wear those puppies at least fifteen times before her hair starts growing in if she wants to make the pain worth it (average cost per wearing: $10.26). Who says writers aren't good mathematicians?

Flynn is a bikini wax devotee herself, too. She actually does the whole thing herself, which perplexes me . . . almost as much as a news story I recently read about a plastic surgeon who performed liposuction on himself. "It's quite entertaining," Flynn promised of her self-stripping.

Shari, forty, was a Brazilian bikini wax virgin before she came to my gym. She had succumbed to the gooey gunk eight years ago, but that was just for a bare-bones, outside-the-lines procedure. It was a family trip to Phoenix a little more than a year ago that prompted her to hop back on the proverbial horse; Flynn was the one who gently persuaded her to go bareback.

There was pain, Shari admitted. About two days' worth. But it was worth it to return home from the locker room and beckon to her husband, "Honey, look what I had done."

"He was like, 'Whoa!'" Shari recalled, which obviously begged my question, "Was it eyes-bug-out *Whoa* or I-want-to-have-sex-right-now *Whoa?*"

Her answer: Probably a combination, but it didn't matter because her virtual vacation to Brazil had left her, um, passport so tender that her hubby might as well have been left stranded at the gate.

Dr. Fisher said this kind of male response is nothing to be surprised by. The hormone dopamine—the same one that skyrockets during a cocaine binge—is driven by pleasure and associated with things that are new, fun, and novel. I guess you could say that a suddenly bare, naked lady, after years of a full bush, can be considered new, fun, and novel. So in a way, a Brazilian bikini wax is the vaginal equivalent to snorting cocaine, only it's legal, it's way less expensive, and it won't burn a hole in your septum!

Regardless, Shari, now a two-finger-strip devotee, said she loves the convenience of getting her bikini line waxed right in the locker room—after all, it is quite a luxury. Even though it can lack confidentiality (you have to check in outside at the athletic desk), there's something to be said for being able to work out, shower, and walk two feet to the aesthetician's room. Shari said she especially likes it for times when she's dropping her children off for tennis or yoga; while the kids are running around, mommy can kill two birds with one $45 stone.

II. Baby's First Razor

There comes a point in every gal's life when she needs a real women's razor. For me, that time came less than a year shy of turning thirty. Why did I wait so long? The answer is an attractive combination of being cheap and stubborn. For five years, I endured cuts the size of Rhode Island on my leg when I shaved with the single-blade blue razors provided in the ladies' locker room, clearly designed for people with hair as thick as pencil refills.

For as long as I used these axe-like tools, I emerged from the shower with marks and slashes of varying degrees decorating my knees, shins, and ankles; my skin resembled the bumper of our poor Mercury Cougar after years of parallel parking in the city. Sometimes the nicks were minor and could be stanched with a piece of tissue; at other times, particularly when I was in a rush, the razor acted as a cheese grater, actually slicing off my skin like a ribbon of Parmesan.

After one particularly angry-looking self-induced mutilation, my husband had had enough. "Why don't you just get some razors made for women?" he asked. "Why keep hurting yourself?"

"Because I'm paying an arm and a leg for my membership—I might as well take advantage of everything I can," I rationalized in my head. But for some reason, my leg being elevated above my head, the only thing that came out was a whiny, "I'm fiiinnne!"

Lo and behold, after Dan returned from his next grocery shopping trip, I found among the cereal and trash bags an eight-pack of pink Venus razors. He bought me pink razors! With *three* blades and swivel heads and rubberized grips and everything. I felt just as special as when he carried me over the threshold (okay, who are we kidding—he steadied me as I tottered and hiccuped my way into the room) on our wedding night.

So I took my new pink babies for a spin the next day at the club. I spread the creamy foam (also compliments of the locker room) all up and down my gams like icing on a birthday cake and went to town.

Instantly, I was transformed into the woman in the commercial, smiling down at mile-long legs as they beaded up with water and begged to be de-fuzzed. As the razor traced my legs like a racecar on a closed track, cutting corners and making turns without kicking up the slightest bit of dust, I felt like a blind person who could see again. Someone who had fallen into a coma before the advent of the Internet and just woken up. That hot-pink razor kissed my ankles instead of chewing

them, caressed my shins like a little pink Fabio. After I rinsed
the residual foam away, my legs were smoother than whipped
cream, thanks to a special moisturizing strip, and there was
not a drop of blood in sight. I even managed to eke out twice
the recommended uses on my first razor and still nary a hair in
site. I had beaten the system. Now, when I walk by those piti-
ful blue razors, lined up in a vertical, wall-mounted stack, I
laugh at the pain I once allowed them to cause me. It's as
if they were the popular high school girls but I, once a bit
dorky, had now blossomed into womanhood.

I Worked Hard for the Money

For about a year during graduate school, I worked as a
cocktail waitress at a trendy bar in Chicago's Lincoln Park. I
begged for Friday and Saturday night shifts because not only
were they the biggest moneymakers, but I was newly single
and hating men, and I intended to stay that way—dateless
and vengeful. So when the weekend came, I would post-
pone my workout until about 8:30 P.M., exercise for an hour,
and then get ready at the health club for my shift, which was
from 10:30 P.M. to 2:30 A.M.

Now when I say get ready, what I really mean is get ready
to make some money. Holy crap, you should've seen the
things I whipped out of my gym bag of tricks. Black mini-
skirts the size of washcloths. Backless tops. Shirts with long,
thin strips of material that wound around my midriff three or
four times, ending in a bow above my navel. And, of course,
the crowd favorite, a pair of black low-rise vinyl pants that I
actually cleaned with Windex. Years later, I would learn that

some of Dan's friends thought I was purposefully trying to dress up like Britney Spears. (This was back in her post-puberty, pre-Cheeto heyday. And no, I was not.)

My makeup routine was elaborate and ritualistic, filled with cat-eyed black liner and lipstick designed to mimic the color your skin takes on after orgasm. I curled my eyelashes and straightened my hair. My body lotion had a hint of shimmer, and I would dust bronzer across my perennially exposed collarbones and waist. I'm sure that some of the late-night exercisers who saw me preparing thought I was a stripper. Not because I had huge fake boobs, but because it was ten o'clock on a Saturday night and I was in the gym locker room wearing knee-high boots that easily made me six foot one and was enveloped in a cloud of perfume that smelled like a mix of candy and sex. They, more appropriately, were wearing sweat-soaked T-shirts and bike shorts. As a defense mechanism, I would always tie my little black apron around my waist to show that yes, I was going to work. I'm not sure why I felt I had something to prove to these strangers, including the locker room's attendants, who looked at me with a combination of confusion and disdain, but I did.

Working out right before my shift had an empowering effect on me. I felt strong and fit, which, in turn, made me feel sexy. And when you're jockeying for tips from a sea of yuppies all dressed in variations of the same striped button-down shirt and black leather jacket, you have to feel sexy . . . and confident. So I guess you could say my weekend beauty ritual was my pep talk for the night. Yet another reason why I loved my locker room. Because remember, as I said before, being at the gym is not just about keeping our hearts healthy—vanity, that deadly sin, is a critical aspect, too.

Once I had my two signature mini-pigtails pulled up in front (I felt the hint of innocence on top balanced out the blatant sexuality below), I was out the door and on my way to work, where my well-planned locker room routine proved well worth it with the clichéd collegiate crowd. My tummy still taut from my workout, I flirted while taking orders from the boys, then made fun of them with the girls at the next table. The male customers loved it when I did shots with them; little did they know I was downing water while they took back harsh vodka. "Ooh!" I would squeal with a little toss of the head. "That's so strong!" Tip, please.

5

Belly Dancing

Learning About Pregnancy
Straight from the Source

One morning as I was dressing to work out, I noticed a gaggle of bobbing bellies assembling in the locker room. I knew something had to be up so I ditched my elliptical machine plans and followed the group down to a studio. Ooh—Pilates for the preggers set! The instructor graciously allowed me to make a quick announcement asking for volunteers for interviews, and, to my delight, every hand shot up. As I dashed around the room to collect phone numbers, all the while dodging rotund tummies and skipping over gurgling babies on blankets, I thanked the women and explained how this would help readers get a first-hand grasp on pregnancy's true impact on body image. That's when I heard somebody shout sarcastically from the corner, "The truth? They can't handle the truth!"

The voice was decidedly feminine, but the Jack Nicholson tone was a bit more *The Shining* than *A Few Good Men*. As it turns out, pregnancy can kick up a wide array of responses concerning body image, from self-loving to self-loathing. It can be something as simple as the way a mother-to-be applies cocoa butter, that purported magical stretch mark elixir: I have seen women lovingly massage the salve into their burgeoning bellies, dreamy smiles spread wide across their faces as nursery rhymes play on their imaginary iPods. I've also seen treadmill queens smear the thick lotion across their stomachs, grimaces firmly in place, as they point out the most minute of markings to their friends and complain about what "this baby" is already doing to their bodies.

Each year, when springtime arrives, pregnant women seem to be blooming everywhere, and my gym is no exception. On the stair-climbers. Lifting weights next to me. In the mommies-to-be aqua class. And, of course, in the locker room. The early ones stretch their T-shirts over their swollen curves until they begin to roll upward at the edges, then switch to more forgiving zip-up sweatshirts and drawstring pants. Some of them continue to work out at an impressive rate, eventually substituting stationary biking, the elliptical machine, and yoga for the riskier kickboxing and running. They waddle purposefully from locker to shower, grab extra white towels to cover their expanding girths, and field advice from the more experienced moms in the bathroom stalls next to them. This is pissing and moaning—literally.

I am the first to admit that I harbor a certain amount of personal fear related to body image and pregnancy. Actually, it's not merely related to body image; it is as completely enmeshed in body image as a chewed-up wad of bubble gum in a little girl's ponytail. My concerns are twofold and, in my opinion, legitimate. First of all, women who have survived an eating disorder and worked through the therapy understand that diseases such as anorexia and bulimia have very much to do with control and very little to do with food. They feel a loss of control over other areas in their lives but, rather conveniently, things such as calories, food, and exercise offer a sense of mastery. Hence, the body becomes a puppet of sorts, the one thing in their lives over which they have power. But when you become pregnant, that power is lost. Breasts develop, the waistline expands, hormones rage, and cravings loom large. I must confess, there's an element of anxiety there for me.

Second, and a bit less selfish, I suppose (or selfless, depending on whether you're a "diaper is half-full" or a "diaper is half-empty" kind of person), is the fear of passing my past concerns about body image on to my child. Suppose I gave birth to a daughter; I could never forgive myself if she grew up to have an eating disorder. Children are incredibly perceptive. Is it so difficult to imagine her watching me eat one type of cheese while I feed her another, or to think of her picking up on a look I might inadvertently give myself in the mirror once in a while? Or her realizing, "Wait, my mom works out a lot but my best friend's mom never works out . . . what's the deal?" And the risk doesn't apply only to daughters; boys are becoming increasingly vulnerable to distorted body image as well.

To be honest, I was shocked—dumbfounded, in fact—when Jane, the woman in my locker room who suffers from profound anorexia, began showing. At first I thought that perhaps she was just bloated, or maybe, thankfully, gaining a few pounds. But it soon became clear that this was baby weight. She was the prototypical example of a bump on two sticks. Jane continued working out with the same fervor, and before long the locker room's whispers confirmed her pregnancy.

How could this be? I was amazed that she was even still menstruating, what with her seeming total lack of body fat. But as her belly grew, Jane stayed on those cardio machines day in and day out, willing her limbs to hold on to their twig-like state. A concerned friend of hers who attended her baby shower told me that when the cake was brought out, she made up an excuse for leaving the room. Fortunately, the baby was born healthy.

It's a little girl.

So it doesn't take a psychology degree to see that for women with body image issues, pregnancy can be a state fraught with concern. To wit: a *New York Magazine* cover story, "The Perfect Pregnancy," focused on women battling the psychological effects of weight gain during pregnancy. The story outed women who spoke of actually wishing for more morning sickness, or of ladies who wore their low maternal weight gain like a Girl Scout badge. (I can picture it now: a pink or blue square patch with a picture of a giant pregnant woman and big red "No" sign encircling her.) And in a society in which maternity mannequins cry out for a pepperoni pizza, in which magazine ads scream, "Motherhood . . . It's HOT!!" and actresses pose for *Playboy* as their newborns snooze off-camera, can we blame them?

But for just as many women, pregnancy can be a respite from an eating disorder or milder body image concerns, and sometimes even a cure. Nada Stotland, MD, a national expert on the psychiatric aspects of women's health, said that although feeling fat during pregnancy is a wildly common sentiment, on the other hand, some women may view it as a time to let down their guard and succumb to their cravings. "They say, 'Finally, now I can eat; I don't have to hold my stomach in all the time,'" she explained.

That's what Abby, twenty-nine, said when she first learned she was pregnant. Ironically, Abby, who exercised thrice weekly, previously had a fairly strong body image, *except* for her abdomen, which she scorned for its stubborn love handles. But once the double lines appeared on her home pregnancy test, she said, she was very happy because she could "just relax and do nothing about it." And by "do nothing," she meant treat her first-trimester nausea with a steady diet of Nachos Bell Grande and Egg McMuffins. "The thought of a fresh fruit or vegetable makes me sick," she said back then. Hello Mickey-D's double cheeseburger and fries. Goodbye broccoli.

Knocked-Up Knockouts

Lauren, thirty-three, didn't just let go of her belly—she puffed it out like a proud peacock for the whole world to see. I first spotted Lauren sitting on the floor of my locker room one morning, breast-feeding her then ten-week-old daughter (she also has a six-year-old). As it turned out, she had just switched to my gym specifically because it offered babysitting services; this way, she could let someone else take care of the baby while she took care of herself.

Unlike women who fret that their early-pregnancy tummies will be mistaken for one too many trips to the ice cream parlor, Lauren would purposely distend her abdomen in the locker room because she hoped somebody would ask whether she was expecting. Later, when she did "pop," Lauren would chat with fellow pregnant locker mates, proudly comparing girths and swapping due dates like so many recipes. She never once felt self-conscious about her pregnant body. On the contrary: "I felt like God! I thought, 'I can *grow* people! I can make people, with *very little help* from anybody else!'" (Imagine SJP from *Sex and the City* saying this and you'll get a more accurate idea of this woman's true amazement over the experience.)

Sure, she realized her body might never be the same again. But, she proposed, who cares? For Lauren, pregnancy changed the way she thinks about her body; she moved away from the aesthetic and into the functional.

"It makes you feel strong and gives you a whole new appreciation for your body as a life-producing source as opposed to something that's just supposed to look thin and sexy." Sure, she has stretch marks, but she earned them. They've become part of the landscape of her body: "They represent two beautiful healthy babies," she said, even though they would typically be considered flaws.

The nine-month journey was a little bit more of a roller coaster ride for thirty-nine-year-old Julie, but nonetheless, she enjoyed the trip tremendously. A circus acrobat, Julie struggled with an eating disorder and body-image issues prior to her pregnancy. Like so many other women, she could look in the mirror and, intellectually, know that she looked spectacularly in shape, but thirty minutes later, that same reflection could bring her down faster than a crashed laptop. This happened not just in the locker room, but in her circus dressing room, too. (She performs a specialized aerial silk act as well as a hand balance routine with her husband-partner.) There was always a feeling that if she could just lose a few more pounds, her act could be that much stronger.

When Julie first found out she was pregnant, she headed straight for her computer and performed two searches. The first was for "athletes and pregnancy" and the second, "pregnancy and eating disorders." She was encouraged to learn that many women with prior eating disorders enjoy very healthy pregnancies. And although the research told her that relapses often happen postpartum, Julie was grateful to be armed with that information.

But what she was even more grateful for was this: While pregnant, Julie had the healthiest body image of her life. It wasn't simply an issue of beauty, she said, but of self-respect. Though she didn't necessarily like the lines of her pregnant body—"I prefer to have a waist," she said dryly—for the first time in her life she was *proud* of how she looked. And that took a lot of the pressure off.

During her last month of pregnancy, while changing out of her sweaty clothes in the locker room, Julie remembers how the standard towel strained to cover her ever-expanding circumference. As she grabbed extras in an attempt to fashion a patchwork towel quilt, a nearby woman made eye contact and smiled. Suddenly, Julie was no longer embarrassed. In her heart, she knew what that smile meant: "I've been there, too." And a sense of camaraderie and delight surged within her as she made her way to the showers, flashing some extra tummy along with her pride.

For some pregnant women, like Barbra, fifty, the concept of baring belly in the locker room was never even an issue. Before the health club phenomenon had even begun, when Jane Fonda was just beginning to market her videos, locker rooms and white towels were for high school football players only. Back then, Barbra got her exercise outdoors, through biking and softball.

But you can take only so many swings until your pregnant belly starts to become a liability. That was the signal for Barbra, then a wispy twenty-five-year-old, to stop playing. But there was no crying in softball. For as the baby grew, she drank up the curvy body that accompanied her pregnancy and stayed after she delivered the first of two children.

"I had hips, a waist, boobs," Barbra said. "I liked the curves. I finally had an adult body."

Alas, her second pregnancy was not so enjoyable. Barbra threw up from conception to delivery, ultimately gaining just 12 or so pounds. But the curves stayed and she rocks them like the Jon Bon Jovi groupie she is. (Note to Jon: Barbra really, really likes you. She even played your music for her two daughters while they were in utero. Please call.)

When "Birth Announcement" Sounds Like "Girth Announcement"

Anne, a thirty-two-year-old mother of two young children, was a self-described "tank" during her last pregnancy who stopped watching the scale once her weight gain hit the 45-pound mark. (She had heard through the grapevine that she should expect to gain from 25 to 35 pounds.) She recalled in vivid detail how a fellow gym-goer, armed with a telltale fake tan and a perky boob job, would prance around the locker room naked, only serving to make Anne feel even bigger. Said Anne without a trace of sarcasm in her voice, "I hated her then and I still do."

During her first pregnancy, Anne eliminated junk food from her diet and was careful to eat a variety of fruits and vegetables. Nonetheless, she said, the pounds piled on, to the point where they were obscuring her vision—not of her toes, but of the pregnancy itself.

"I'd call my husband after the doctor's appointment and tell him how many pounds I'd gained," she recalled, "and he'd ask, 'Well, how's the baby?' In hindsight, it is sad that my husband had to keep our perspective, [pointing out things like] the doctor said the baby's heartbeat was good."

About halfway through her pregnancy, Anne gave up on working out because she was embarrassed to be seen at the gym. And because of this, she confessed, she felt like a failure.

Today, to the casual observer, Anne appears to be a trim, petite woman. But no, she assured me. Naked, pregnancy has made her look as if she should be in *National Geographic,* with "everything down, swinging." Glancing back today, she curses all the time and energy she spent worrying about her thighs; now, the body image issue du jour is her skin, which, like a stretched-out rubber band, never regained its elasticity. Sadly, she finds herself tensing up when her husband cuddles behind her in bed because she feels as if her stomach and breasts are "lying on the bed" next to her. Anne fears she will not have another child because she is so uncomfortable with the effects pregnancy has had on her physique.

For Kelly, too, pregnancy inflicted such emotional turmoil on her body image that she's considering not having another child because of it. Though never diagnosed with an eating disorder, the thirty-five-year-old has always struggled with body image concerns, working out five or six times a week and painstakingly watching her food intake. When she learned she was pregnant, that behavior only intensified, especially in the beginning when she was caught in belly purgatory, that in-between stage of looking "big" but not yet looking obviously pregnant.

"I was so petrified of gaining too much weight, I probably weighed myself every day," Kelly confessed. "A lot of my friends said I would gain 40 pounds and so I should just eat what I wanted and enjoy it." But Kelly was dead set against handing her hard-earned physique over to Mother Nature. She wanted to beat the odds. However, she was frustrated with working out and eating properly and still seeing her body growing bigger and bigger every day—even if it was the *baby* that was doing the growing.

Of her experience in the locker room, Kelly said that being pregnant made an already uncomfortable experience even worse. She even used a private changing area: "There was no way I would show my stomach to anybody. I just felt like people were staring at me. It wasn't the way I wanted to look." Meanwhile, Kelly found herself looking at other pregnant women in the locker room and thinking, "Wow, they look really good" or "She's really small."

At month five, Kelly's obstetrician was unhappy with her low weight gain and told her to start putting on some more pounds. Eventually, she wound up delivering a healthy baby girl, and quickly lost the 28 pounds she had gained. She did, however, put some weight back on, a result of the hectic new-mother schedule that has prevented her from working out as much as she would have liked. "That's why," she admitted, "I struggle with thinking about having another one."

Ultimately, the decision over the amount of weight you gain may be out of your hands. The American College of Obstetricians and Gynecologists (ACOG) recommends a gain of from 25 to 35 pounds for women of normal weight; from 28 to 40 pounds for underweight women; and from 15 to 25 pounds for overweight women. But, as women like Anne and Kelly often find out, ACOG ain't you, and ACOG ain't the one waking up with a 1:00 A.M. craving for buffalo wings smothered in blue cheese.

Dr. Stotland, the psychiatrist quoted earlier, said recommendations have changed over the centuries, so much so that when her mother was pregnant with her, severe diet restriction was in vogue. In fact, her mother's ob/gyn threatened to bar patients from his practice if they gained more than his recommended number. (I would bet good money this doctor also had a small penis, but it's not nice to talk about people you don't know.) But, as Dr. Stotland pointed out, the pendulum swings, and standards have relaxed. Nonetheless, she noted that "if you gain a lot, you have to get rid of it, and that takes effort."

Breasts: They Do a Body Good

Which brings us to breast-feeding, that legendary calorie-torching, baby-nourishing, mother-bonding miracle.

Kelly chose to breast-feed and said the 28 pounds melted off. Lauren, the woman I met while she was nursing in our locker room, said breast-feeding surely had its metabolic benefits, but that was in no way the deciding factor in her decision. "Nursing a child makes you appreciate the fact these are really here for a purpose," she said about her breasts. In acknowledgment of women who want to breast-feed but are unable to, Lauren said she feels especially thankful for having nursed: "I was able to grow the baby on the inside for nine months and then continue to grow the baby on the outside. It makes the birthing process somehow less traumatic. In terms of how I view my breasts, I care a lot less how they look and care a lot more about what they can do."

Speaking of how they look, Lauren had some colorful descriptions for the changes her breasts went through during pregnancy. "You look like a porn star," she exclaimed, looking down in awe at her chest, still in disbelief. "They're hard as rocks and engorged with milk. When I wake up in the morning, they're these huge melons." Nursing catapulted Lauren, typically in the C to D range, into "the vowels."

But although incredibly rewarding, nursing is not for the faint of heart, Lauren said. "If you're going to breast-feed your child, you have to get comfortable whipping out your boobs wherever you happen to be." Luckily, Lauren is.

But what she can't get over is other women's reactions to her breast-feeding. Lauren remains incredulous that gym members can handle seeing naked women of all ages sashaying through the locker room, yet they risk whiplash to avoid making eye-to-nipple contact as she feeds her child. She finds it hysterically nonsensical, like a brain surgeon who's afraid of a little eye crust. So she said it's especially nice when other women stop and offer support or share stories. These women, Lauren said, tend almost exclusively to be moms who have previously breast-fed, or at least are comfortable with the concept. In fact, she said, just the other day, an older woman saw her on the floor and said, "Jeez, you'd think they could put out a couch. The guys have a plasma screen TV in their locker room." (In our manager's defense, the women's locker room *did* just receive a similar overhaul.)

Deflated Egos

For many women, the most shocking pregnancy-related jolt occurs after breast-feeding, and can most tidily be summed up by Jill, forty-one, who now self-deprecatingly describes herself as "a nipple on a bone."

Jill worked out diligently during her pregnancies. For instance, she pulled one child in a bike buggy to the health club (thirteen miles roundtrip!), exercising *more* at the gym while pregnant with her second child. She managed to keep her weight gain to only 22 pounds: "There was no way I was going to put myself in a position where I'd have to lose 50 pounds [after delivery]," she said. She feels that breast-feeding was pushed on her, and although she acknowledged its health benefits for the baby, she believes the toll it takes on the mother is not only unacknowledged, it's downright ignored. So much so that, after weaning her second baby, she actually went in for a consultation with a plastic surgeon for a possible breast augmentation.

"I had looked in the mirror and I was devastated," Jill described. "I felt worse about my body than ever before." She went so far as to begin wearing a bra under her sports bra for added padding while working out—a getup that sounds about as comfortable as going without socks in faux-leather loafers on a hot afternoon, or wearing your skinny jeans on your worst PMS day. Ultimately, though, she decided against the implants.

"I realized I'd have to wait until my child was big enough to get into bed on her own," she said, alluding to the fact that surgery would prevent her from heavy lifting. "As time went on, I started to think, 'Is it worth it to put myself at risk just for vanity?' Now, I look at my children and think, 'Who would raise them if something happened to me?'" So Jill has instead amassed an impressive collection of padded bras and in the meantime is hoping the athletic-wear industry will design a line of padded workout gear for women like her. "There are a ton of women who feel like this," she said. "It's not right we should have to feel so self-conscious."

Tracie, a thirty-four-four-year-old mother of two who used her gym's pool to ease the weight of her pregnancy belly, never considered having plastic surgery. But that didn't stop her from hitting a lingerie shop popular with the local breast cancer community for their comforting demeanor and wide assortment of bra inserts and moldings.

"I loved my boobs when I was pregnant," Tracie said. "I felt like, *I am woman!*' But afterward, I thought people were going to think I had had a mastectomy," because she had lost so much breast tissue. In the store, there was a woman in the dressing room next to her who was in her final round of chemotherapy; they were both having the same inserts put into their bathing suits. Tracie admitted she felt like a brat: "But I couldn't help it. I felt like less of a woman. I thought, 'Is my husband going to feel like he got a raw deal?'"

This was a common sentiment mentioned by many women—the notion that their after-delivery bodies had somehow let their husbands down. Anne said that whereas her husband used to be "a boob guy," now it's a no-fly zone. She has simply rendered it off-limits for foreplay.

When she had finished nursing, Michelle, thirty-eight, approached her body with the same gusto and vigor of which many of the women I interviewed spoke: She wanted to get rid of it. After breast-feeding her first child for fourteen months and her second for eighteen months, this knockout brunette watched her naturally full Cs deflate until there was nothing left. (The connective tissue that supports breasts, as well as the skin itself, expands during pregnancy and lactation, then shrinks afterward.) Although she loved the experience of breast-feeding and said she wouldn't change it for the world, Michelle, an active woman who works out regularly, felt her self-esteem take a hit as her breasts shrank. In the locker room, she changed quickly and self-consciously; she lost her sexual confidence with her husband (she's now divorced).

So Michelle sought a breast augmentation. The surgery restored her breasts to a 36C. Now, in the locker room, she thinks her breasts look great—even more so when compared to those around her. "I see women my age or up who obviously have had children [and they have] flat, saggy boobs like I had and I think, 'Oh my God, I wonder if that bothers them?'"

The augmentation has boosted her self-esteem in places besides the locker room; flattering comments continually stream in regarding her physique. But it's never enough for people, from strangers to her boyfriend, simply to say, "You look great." There's always the addendum ". . . for someone with two kids." Not that she minds. Michelle is back to her former bombshell status and she enjoys a healthy sex life. And her younger sister has followed in her stroller tracks: She, too, has just had breast implants put in, following the nursing of her own two children.

From Nice Jewish Girl to the Virgin Mary

It was a bright, sunny day in late April when I suddenly became nine months pregnant. It's not something we had planned. I'm religious about my birth control. But it was something that needed to happen. After all, how could I write meaningfully about pregnancy and body image if I had never had any sort of bun in my oven? And so we did it. The old, old, old-fashioned way. The Virgin Mary way. The Empathy Belly® Pregnancy Simulator way.

The Empathy Belly is an educational tool often used in high school sex-ed courses and childbirthing classes to mimic the feeling of a full-term pregnancy. Strapped on like a backward-facing vest and secured with Velcro straps, the device gets you (or the man in your life) as damn close as possible to being a full nine months as anything else. That is, except for a backpack stuffed with 25 pounds of kitty litter, which a colleague told me she used in her Lamaze class years ago because the costly Empathy Belly was out of their budget. (Coincidentally, her son has an uncanny ability to lap up milk from his cereal bowl and loves being rescued from trees by firefighters.)

When I finally got my hands on the magical belly, I felt like a kid in a candy store. I unzipped the duffel bag and found what looked like a life-sized pregnant doll torso, a circular blue vinyl bag (the bladder), a funnel, two extremely heavy, baseball-sized metal orbs, a sandbag, and a strap, which I would soon learn was used to constrict breathing. Following the instructions, I used the funnel to fill the abdomen with fifteen cups of warm water (to give the sensation of amniotic fluid), and inserted the weighted balls and sandbag into their proper compartments. My husband helped me hoist the contraption on and, save for a near eye-gouging with my giant, cone-shaped pregnancy boobs, he safely strapped me in.

Wait! What was that? "I think I felt the baby kicking," I exclaimed incredulously. Dan stared at me as if I were crazy. But yes, I had felt something—a small hard ball floating in the bladder was "kicking" me every time I moved.

Together, we moved to the bathroom mirror to take a look. Gazing back at me was Robin Williams in preparation for his role in *Mrs. Doubtfire,* the movie about the cross-dressing nanny. This would not work. I needed some cute maternity clothes, but somehow, I didn't think my little satin cami with the built-in cups was going to cut it.

However, as it turns out, my sartorial inclinations were right in line with what Dr. Stotland said has been a radical change in the public display of pregnancy over the last few years.

"It's very striking," she said. "Things like uncovered pregnancy bellies or clothes that are just stretched over and not roomy . . . convey a message of acceptance and pride. In that sense it should be easier for women to live with that body image."

Unfortunately, I had just loaned my backless, navel-cut maternity halter top to a friend, so my hubby fished me out the biggest shirt he owned, a maroon tee from his mortgage company's softball league. All of a sudden, I was a big, blobby walking advertisement with no shape or definition—just one diagonal line from my neck to my navel. But with these new knockers, I wanted, and needed, lift and separation. I tried tucking in some material beneath my breasts, then fitting the rest around the belly. The final step: tying a cute little knot in the back in the style of a teen pop star.

Before hitting the gym, I decided to take a walk around the neighborhood and test the tummy out. About a minute into my stroll, a man in a truck honked at me. I struggled as the pregnant angel on my left shoulder screamed, "Hey, sicko, lady with a baby in here!" and the skinny devil on my right snickered, "Yeah, you still got it, Toots."

I walked a few blocks to the home of my friend Veronica, who has a seven-year-old son. She took one look at my belly and proclaimed, "You're way too high. There's no way any-one would believe you're nine months pregnant."

"I haven't dropped yet, bitch!" I snapped back at her. Okay, calm down, I told myself. I wasn't *really* pregnant, wasn't privy to the hormone-addled attitude.

After we had chatted for a bit, I left, bumping my belly on her iron gate. On the way home, caressing my fake abdomen while holding my back for support, the first benefit of preg-nancy kicked in: The ice cream man offered me a free cone. I politely declined, but inside I was loving the treatment. Next, two teenagers walked by, one of them wearing a shirt that so eloquently proclaimed, "Let the fucking begin." I glared at him with evil eyes, telepathically conveying the message, "That's what got me here, prick."

Belly Goes to the Gym

Later that afternoon, I pulled on a pair of cute heather gray shorts and a sports bra and got Belly ready for a trip to the health club. As we walked into the locker room, we were greeted by—I kid you not—a completely naked redhead standing before the mirror, clipping her fingernails. It's a good thing my first trimester nausea was long gone because the fragments of this woman's nails were shooting off in var-ious directions and a thumbnail went whizzing by my head. Was this really the type of environment I wanted my child to be raised in?

I had to pee badly, what with the little ball pounding on my bladder, so I shuffled off to the bathroom, extremely self-conscious of the tent-like silhouette that seemed to confront me at every turn. Head-on, I looked exactly the same, but from the side, I was a house. My lower half looked ridiculously small, almost bird-like in comparison.

I chose the smallest bathroom stall in which to test myself. Not smart. As I assumed my favored squat-and-hover position in the already-cramped quarters, I quickly found I couldn't even see the toilet seat because my belly blocked my view. Clearly, my aim was going to be somewhat of a crapshoot. And then, as I let my full bladder release into a state of what would usually be pure bliss, I realized something: I still had to pee! Even at the end. With my thighs quaking from supporting the extra weight and a single bead of sweat rolling down my forehead, the automatic flush activated, taunting me with its premature swoosh. I stood up and emerged from the stall, wholly unsatisfied with the transaction that had just occurred and sure I'd be back sooner than I had hoped.

Making my way up the stairs to the stretching area, I saw two teenaged training assistants with whom I'm friendly. Their eyes practically bungee-jumped from their sockets. So cute, those teenage boys with little to no sex education from the schools! As I watched the other non-pregnant women around me, I felt uncomfortable in my own "skin" because they seemed to have so much more freedom of movement. Whereas I waddled, they ran. I struggled to fit into the leg adductor; they slipped into the hamstring machine with ease. I must admit, though, I did catch a few sidelong glances that seemed, ahem, pregnant with envy. Perhaps these women were trying to conceive, or had been aching for a baby for a while, but some of those looks definitely indicated that their owners wanted my bump.

I walked around the track—one lap—and it seemed to take forever. By the end, I was holding my back for support for real and was grumpy from being passed by so many joggers.

A bright spot: Two male friends who were in on my experiment told me I would make a cute pregnant lady. But by that point, I couldn't care less about my M.I.L.F. factor; I just wanted this contraption off. Yes, I had that luxury, and I took advantage of it. Belly came off, and I returned to my locker to change into my fitted UW T-shirt. Grabbing a magazine and heading back to work out, I checked my profile in the mirror and was surprised to find myself looking so . . . flat. In fact, I looked fairly boyish. I suppose I *had* enjoyed certain aspects of the voluptuousness of my belly and boobs, even if they were accompanied by an aching back and made walking down stairs downright lethal.

I guess the Empathy Belly had achieved its goal: It made me feel more empathy for the daily plight of pregnant women, and it also gave me at least the smallest inkling of how pregnancy affects a woman's body image. At the end of the day, I definitely felt I had experienced something special and unique.

But I also took my birth control pill, and right on time.

6

Pimples, Crotches, and Butts, Oh My!

Locker Room Nudity in All Its Splendor . . . and Horror

I'm not exactly what you'd call a shrinking violet. Never have been. I've been known to hug the mailman when a big check arrived, break out into my Britney Spears routine in the middle of the supermarket, and talk to complete strangers about their cervixes. Sometimes, people respond; other times, they back away. Slowly. No bother. It's who I am, love me or leave me.

When it comes to public displays of nudity, I was recently thrust into the spotlight—literally—when my mother and I embarked on the marathon process of shopping for a wedding dress. The last time my mom saw me fully naked was probably when I was in elementary school. But, as any bride-to-be will tell you, when you're trying on wedding gowns, modesty falls somewhere on the list of priorities between chair coverings and feeding the band. So I figured, "Hey, if

Ethel, the Brides 'R' Us fitting specialist, can see my boobies, so can my mom."

As the gowns started piling up in my dressing room, I was told to start trying on anything that caught my eye. With my poor little five-foot-three mom becoming more and more obscured by the tower of satin and silk, I began the somewhat bizarre process of removing my jeans, top, and bra in front of the woman who had wiped my cutely dimpled tush when I was a toddler but had never seen it with real-woman dimples of cellulite. Her reaction?

"You're wearing a thong?! Oh my God, Leslie. How can you wear those things? They go right up your butt!"

"Um, yeah, Mom. That's kind of the point. They're designed to go up your butt and stay there, so you don't have panty lines and don't have to keep picking a wad of scrunched-up panty material out of your crack." Which, of course, is where normal underwear inevitably winds up migrating on me.

Regardless, the mother-daughter nakedness barrier had been sufficiently broken. We ultimately found the dress, and Mom continued to see me naked until the day of the wedding, when she was joined by seven bridesmaids who witnessed me in all my stomach-crunched, spray-tanned glory as I stepped into the gown of my dreams. Wearing nothing but a lacy white thong.

My advice: If you ever want a quick-and-dirty introduction to being naked in front of other people, visit a public dressing room. It could be a bridal salon, a department store bra fitting, or one of those communal dressing areas that didn't shell out the bucks for doors on the stalls. You'll get over your fear of public nudity *real* fast. Trust me.

Which brings us to the locker room.

When I had my eating disorder, I was ashamed of my naked body; but now when it comes to being naked in the locker room, my extroverted personality has served me well in my recovery. I am able to take a more laissez faire approach: I don't change in the bathroom stall. I don't hurry to put my clothes on with water still running down my back. On the other hand, I don't "air dry," à la Cuba Gooding, Jr., in *Jerry McGuire*. Rather, I wait, towel strategically placed, until my skin is more or less dry to the touch. And once appropriately silky and fruity-scented, I'm not afraid to pull on my G-string in full view (as opposed to the supremely popular, modesty-preserving version of tugging one's underwear up with a towel wrapped around the waist, then letting the towel fall to the floor and quickly hopping into a pair of pants.)

Mind you, I do not strut about the locker room naked. Ever. This seems both nightmarish and obnoxious to me. As with sunbathing, the farthest I'll go is topless. However, there are many women in my locker room who do choose to walk around in various stages of undress; they range from the most modest (towel around the waist, towel around the chest) to the most brazen ("Towel? You mean the thing I dry my dishes with?") This latter category tends to be the same women who sit bare-assed on the benches as they work the knots out of their hair with the communal Barbasol-soaked combs or pick the paint chips from their toenail polish.

Most women fall somewhere in between: They opt for some sort of below-the-waist coverage and a towel draped around the neck to obscure each breast but allow the back and stomach to air out. I call this "The Rocky," and it seems to be the uniform of choice among women ages twenty to sixty. In my research, I noticed most teenagers were still a bit skittish, favoring secure single-towel coverage around the chest (The Rocky can swing to and fro, and is therefore prone to possible wardrobe malfunctions), but much older women seem to have pretty much accepted their bodies and tend not to rely on towels as security blankets. These free birds strip out of their workout gear and saunter to the showers, towel in hand as if it were merely the latest Hermès bag to hit the stores.

The Full Monty

I couldn't help but laugh out loud when I stumbled across the following blog entry on Hissyfit.com, written by Tara Ariano:

> There's this one woman in particular at my gym who is probably fifty. And in the time it takes me to leave the shower, put on all my clothes, finish my ablutions, and leave the room with all my gear, she'll spend fully nude, just going to town with a bottle of Vaseline Intensive Care on every inch of her exposed skin. Which is every inch of skin on her body. Oh, and also? She wears thongs. And not just regular, businesslike thongs from, like, Gap, but crazy sex thongs with way too many straps and elastics and pulleys and whatnot.

This rant captures the essence of "The Full Monty." Not that I have a problem with keeping my skin supple or donning racy thongs—I even have a few sassy numbers myself, including a little black mesh pair with a dangling gold dollar bill charm, which I like to wear in Las Vegas, and a see-through lacy pink one, which, for no explicable reason whatsoever, has a frilly patch sewn on that says, "But I Like You."

Still, strut around in them in front of other women at my health club? No thanks.

I have seen these women who choose the locker room to conduct their own sort of self-care modus operandi. With loving strokes, they tenderly and carefully rub apricot-scented lotion into each limb, then switch to a heavier lavender-perfumed cream for their hands and feet. They might apply a facial masque and patiently wait for the dark aqua gel to dry to a cracked light blue. All the while, they're nude. Not just turned around, facing the locker, mind-my-own-business nude. We're talking legs-splayed, moan-and-groan, "God, I deserve to pamper myself like this" butt naked.

I called the blog writer, Tara, who is thirty-one, to inquire a bit further about her experiences with nudity in the locker room. As it should happen, she told me, just the other day, there was a woman blow-drying her hair and putting on a full face of makeup—sitting down, completely in the buff. "If women are that relaxed about their body image, God bless 'em," Tara commented, "but there's a line between self-confidence and hygiene. Even though they did just replace the seats in front of the vanity, I feel doing your makeup in the nude on a chair is on the wrong side of the line."

And then there is the young and apparently very flexible woman who, I have it on good authority, makes it a habit to stretch on the floor of the locker room. Naked. The kind of ballet stretch in which your left leg points west and your right leg points east and you bend at the waist, touching your toes with your opposing arm. Talk about being on the wrong side of the line—this girl straddles it like a ballerina-turned-stripper.

Of course, it's not always a matter of showing off. Sometimes you have to be nude simply out of necessity. After all, it is a *locker room*. It's not as if the women who walk around without clothes on are doing so in a convenience store or a court of law. But you can find ways to be discreet about it, if you so choose.

Take, for instance, my friend Amanda, who, when changing or going to toss a towel in the dirty-laundry bin, employs a technique she likes to call "The Crabwalk." It's a move similar to the one so many of us have used in the boudoir: We need to get up from a bed with a man in it and go to the bathroom, but we don't want our backsides to be visible (even though we trusted the man in the bed enough to be intimate with him).

Moving sideways, slowly but stealthily, only allowing her front side to show, Amanda feels secure enough to make her way from her locker to the towel bin and back, sans towel.

"It's all about the crabwalk," Amanda assured me one night, slightly tipsy from an evening of Merlot. Left foot across right. Repeat. "I don't want people to see any imperfections back there. The front side of me is much better than the back side." I called her the next day for a sober confirmation and her position remained firm: Wine or no wine, crab is where it's at.

For Kasia, the woman whose glimpse of another woman's *Maxim*-like breasts set off a whole slew of reactions, changing out in the open is a refreshing change of pace. "It's the only opportunity we really have to see what other women's nude or seminude bodies actually look like up close and personal, given that most of women's exposure to other women's bodies are in magazines, TV, and movies, where things have been stretched and airbrushed and Photoshopped and tinted to unrealistic perfection," she said. Kasia acknowledged that her attitude might seem a bit out of the ordinary, considering her intense reaction to that ridiculously augmented woman and that she continues to struggle with body-image problems. But still, she finds it "ridiculous" when some women retreat to the locker room's toilet stalls to change. "A huge part of me believes that we will never achieve self-acceptance until we all stop hiding from each other."

Sometimes, it can be a matter of life or death that forces us to confront our feelings about displays of nudity in the locker room. Barb, fifty, was taking a shower when she heard cries for help coming from the Jacuzzi area. She peered out just in time to see an overheated woman passing out and falling to the floor. The woman's daughter, maybe twenty-seven or twenty-eight, frantically tried to cover her mother's naked body; Barb, also nude, dropped to the floor in an attempt to help the woman's mother.

With the paramedics on the way, the woman soon regained consciousness, apparently mortified to have been in such a compromised position. But although Barb could understand that, what she could not understand was the reaction of the crowd who looked on as she tried to administer help.

"People were all aghast that I was naked, bringing robes for us," she remembered. "It's like the nudity was more horrific than her condition." I asked Barb whether, during the ordeal, it had entered her mind to take a minute to cover up. Her answer: "Not once."

"I don't know why I'm so comfortable [with nudity]," explained Barb, a middle school counselor who was raised in a Catholic family. Most women, she has noticed, cannot even speak to one another in the locker room if they are naked. "I think it comes later in life. It stems not only from body image, but from whether you are unconditional in your love for yourself."

Hide and Go "Eek"

On the other end of the skin-baring spectrum are those women who are seemingly able to disrobe and get dressed again in the blink of an eye. These ladies have an almost Svengali-like ability to go from turban and towel to jeans and a sweater in less time than I can shout, "Wait, I dropped a contact. Nobody move!" Move? Please. They've already hightailed it to their cars and are on their way home.

I once saw a woman dressed in jeans, heels, and a black bra, but with a towel wrapped around her chest, applying her makeup and styling her hair. I have a difficult time understanding the purpose of this get-up. Was she self-conscious about her belly? Or just extremely modest? Because if either is true, then why not just put on a shirt and be done with it?

I guess that even in a world where a sexy desperate housewife can cause a nationwide uproar by dropping her towel in a men's locker room on TV, but ultimately be redeemed by the Federal Communications Commission as decent and dandy, women with more than a modicum of modesty do still exist.

Debbie, thirty-five, belongs to this group of women, who from here on out I will refer to as the "Thoroughly Modest Millies." She subscribes to the YMCA's locker room philosophy, "Less Thongs, More Flip-Flops." For Debbie, nudity is more of a private experience, not something to be trotted around the locker room like the latest pair of designer sneakers. Women who blow-dry their hair topless irk her to no end. Much like the government's case for stomping out smoking in public restaurants, Debbie views topless grooming as robbing her of her right to breathe boob-free air.

"Why are you standing there in front of the mirror without a top on?" she asked of no one in particular when I posed the nudity question to her. "Put a bra on! Cover up your private parts. To me, that's personal and private. I don't understand how people can just walk around and show everybody everything. Plus, it's never the saggy-boobed fat women. [No really, Debbie. Tell us what you really think.] It's the women with the great bodies." It turns out that Debbie would rather see a woman in a bra and panties, with no towel, than a topless woman with a towel wrapped around her waist.

To me, this seems crazily foreign. A woman in a bra and panties in the mirror next to me, especially one with a nice figure, would trigger a sense of competition. Somehow, the presence of the towel makes it more clinical and detached, regardless of how nice the boobs/stomach/legs that are showing.

As it turns out, Debbie may be on to something when it comes to her admonishing my seminude blow-drying. Lillian Glass, PhD, the Beverly Hills body-language expert and psychologist, explained to me that modesty is innately ingrained in humans. It's just that in some people *(c'est moi?),* this trait goes unchecked or expresses itself at different levels. Certain women, Dr. Glass said, flaunt what their mommas gave 'em. Unfortunately, this may not be very comforting to other women, even those with the best of bods, let alone those who feel self-conscious in the locker room.

Debbie admitted that she walks around naked after she showers at home, so she considered the fact that perhaps some women truly consider the locker room an extension of the house. But she also acknowledged that her discomfort with nudity in the locker room may actually be masked jealousy—not just of their bodies, but of their mind-set, their confidence.

Twenty-three-year-old Lauren described her Thoroughly Modest Millie status as having even deeper roots. When she was growing up, her uncle, who was mentally handicapped, lived with the family. For the female members of her household, that meant constantly being aware of things such as open doors and a possible lack of privacy. Combined with a family that simply never changed in front of one another, that has translated into Lauren's feelings of uneasiness with locker room nudity. After showering, she usually dries off, wraps the towel around her chest, puts her bra on *over* the towel, and then pulls the towel out.

"If other people are naked, it doesn't bother me, but I just wouldn't do it," she said. "I'm not a shy person [in everyday life], but as far being naked goes, not so much. I'm just not someone who can completely forget about it." And, Lauren explained, she doesn't want to make those around her feel uncomfortable.

Changing the Way We Change

Then there are the women who started off one way—typically as Thoroughly Modest Millies—but have broken out of the cocoon of modesty and made their way to the other side. The naked butterfly side. Take Tina, thirty, for example. As a teenager, Tina was not very active. But as she approached her twenties, she picked up swimming. The sport transformed her body, but still she found herself showering in her swimsuit, then scurrying to a private area to change.

That is, until a seventy-seven-year-old fellow swimmer came along and altered Tina's self-perception for the better. Tina soon struck up a friendship with the grandmother in the purple swim cap who would peel off her wet bathing suit free from fear of prying eyes. Meanwhile, Tina shampooed her hair nearby, still clad in her one-piece.

"I began to think, 'Why am I afraid of taking off my bathing suit?'" Tina remembered aloud. This older woman, whose body was covered with a map of wrinkles and sags, was comfortable chatting openly in the nude. So why couldn't an in-shape, youthfully blessed Tina enjoy the same freedom? That was her turning point. Now, she said, "It's all nudity, all the time." In the locker room, that is.

For Kate, twenty-four, the process has taken about five years, but the results have been extraordinary. In high school and the beginning of college, she recalls herself as being extremely self-conscious—to the point where she wouldn't even want her boyfriend to see her naked, let alone a bunch of strangers in a locker room. But as she began taking women's education courses at her university, things began to click. She would think back to her childhood, where being naked was considered healthy and normal in her family. She was a lifelong soccer player, and instead of craving the "long, skinny legs" of, say, a ballet dancer, she gradually began to appreciate her athletic figure. Pretty soon, she said, "I wasn't afraid to be nude."

You can say that again. Now Kate and her mom hit the gym together and afterward sink into the hot tub, no bathing suits—no anything, for that matter. She admitted a lot of people think the relationship is weird. "But my mom works out a lot, she's in pretty good shape, she eats well. That will hopefully be what I look like when I'm her age." Kate spoke with an air of knowledge rarely heard in a woman in her early twenties, and I must admit, I'm a bit jealous of her level of body acceptance at such a young age. She has found her comfort level far earlier than many women and because of that, the locker room is no longer a scary place for her.

Dorrie, forty-three, used to be so anxious in the locker room that she would duck into the club's private changing room to get undressed: "My friends thought I was nuts. They'd say, 'There she goes again, into the changing room.'" Dorrie isn't sure why it was so painful for her to be naked in front of her friends and coworkers, but believes it was these same women who helped draw her out of those closed-off quarters five or six years ago. Some of them are the teachers she works with; others are women she's seen over and over at the health club. But all of them are outgoing, and their easygoing attitude rubbed off on Dorrie, even through the wooden door.

As she went to the club more and more, Dorrie grew more secure and relaxed with shedding her clothes out in the open—but she does so at rapid-fire speed, quickly changing into a bra and underwear. She always picks the same locker, one close to the showers, out of sight of the mirrors. When other women walk around naked, Dorrie still feels on edge, mostly because "you don't know where to look." A downward glance makes you a pervert; a straightforward, eye-to-eye glare makes you seem like a robot.

Still, these have been big steps for this once-beyond Thoroughly Modest Millie. Dorrie is to be congratulated, for she has, quite literally, come out of the closet.

Rejected Letters to *Penthouse,*
Part I: Twins

I don't recall the first time I laid eyes on Mary and Maureen, identical twins, in my health club, but I remember thinking they were beautiful. Tall, with long legs and great breasts, the pair was well known and well liked throughout my gym, even if they were quite often impossible to tell apart. These talkative teachers with curly brunette hair were quite popular with the men in the weight room, many of whom I'm sure carried that time-honored mental torch held especially for twins, but Mary and Maureen had lots of female friends, too. People were simply drawn to them.

I was one of those people. I've always found twins fascinating, but these two were just so friendly and outgoing that you couldn't help but want to be near them. We'd often talk in the locker room, and when our conversations eventually wound down, our sweaty clothes would be uncomfortable and stripping time would come. And as these thirty-six-year-old sisters started to change for the showers, I would find myself wondering whether it was weird to be naked in front of your twin sister or whether it was a built-in body image bonus. After all, we singletons have our imaginations to carry us away into Perceived Flaw Land, but identical twins have a living, breathing replica staring them right in the face. So I asked them: Naked twin—bane or boon?

Both agreed that having a locker room doppelganger is definitely a bonus. "It keeps me in check," Maureen said. "I look at Mary and think, 'She looks great, so that's how I must look. Or if she looks like she's gained a little weight, I think, 'Is that how I look?'" Their shared DNA serves as an instant mirror, a constant check that tells them, "OK, I look ____ today." (Maureen even recalled looking at her sister's legs and thinking the words, "*Our* legs are getting fat." Not "*Her* legs," but "*Our* legs.")

Mary said having a twin comes in especially handy when dealing with their "trouble area," their stomachs. Maureen, Mary said, has always been five pounds thinner, but nonetheless, the belly is where they both store their extra weight. So whereas they might feel self-conscious about asking a friend whether their bellies look big, they can always count on one another for blunt honesty. The result: They motivate each other to eat healthfully, they work out together, and they see the results, both naked and clothed.

As far as locker room nudity, they aren't quick to dress, but they don't loll around naked, either. They wear towels to and from the showers. There are few parts of each other's bodies they haven't taken a good, hard look at. Mary and Maureen tend to not compare their bodies with those of other women at the gym because in their minds, what's the point? The only truly accurate comparison would be with each other because, as Maureen pointed out, "other women are not an accurate gauge."

This notion takes me by surprise; it makes so much sense that it seems silly not to have thought of it before. It almost seems like *the* cure to woes about body image, tied neatly in a package. But how could other women put it into play for themselves? That is, how could we stop comparing ourselves to each other when every other body is different from our own, and we are the only one with our belly, our ass, our legs? This would require a sea change in our way of thinking, but then again, isn't that what this book is calling for? An entire re-imagining of the "perfect" body, one that uses our *own* body as the gauge by which we measure ourselves?

Rejected Letters to *Penthouse,*
Part II: The Shower

One of my favorite memories of the locker room, one that always brings a smile to my face when I think of it, features my friend Randi. We were engaged in a deep conversation about her former boyfriend, who couldn't get it up, emotionally speaking. I was on a time schedule, so the talk needed to be carried over to the shower. Just as I was about to gather up my toiletries, though, it came to my attention that, horror of horrors, I had forgotten my flip-flops. (Tennis ace Serena Williams has publicly admitted to wearing Kate Spade shower sandals in her locker room. My flip-flops have hula girls on them and cost $3. To each her own.)

Anyone who knows me knows that I can be a hypochondriac to the umpteenth degree, mistaking slightly swollen glands for mono and night sweats for cancer. Not so long ago, during a particularly dark period in my life, I even convinced myself, and I do mean *truly* convinced myself, that I had Parkinson's disease, when it turns out what I really had was an anxiety disorder that caused my hands to tremble. So you can see how going barefoot in a public shower was out of the question. I shudder to think what lurks in those tiles and crevices.

So I, an adult woman with a master's degree, came up with the brilliant idea of showering in my socks. Those 100 percent cotton puppies would definitely keep the germs at bay, right? So off I padded to the shower, Randi in tow, the two of us talking the whole time as if this were a completely normal scenario.

Here's where it gets steamy: I turned on the shower, tested the temperature, and stepped into the private stall, leaving the curtain open so that Randi and I could continue our discussion face-to-face. I was essentially 100 percent naked, shampooing my hair, soaping up my body, and letting those bubbles run down my curves; it was as if I were in a porn scene, and Randi was watching my every move. Hot, right? Except for the fact that I was wearing soggy, disgusting little athletic socks. At one point, when I lifted my right leg up to shave, I looked at Randi and said, "You know, this would be every guy's fantasy, right?" We looked at my socks and burst out laughing. A classic bonding moment.

Germ Warfare

That little X-rated story, depending on whether you're a Full Monty or a Thoroughly Modest Millie, either tickles or horrifies you. Regardless, it provides a perfect segue into a little-talked-about aspect of locker room culture that is tied into certain aspects of modesty and that can be tidily summed up in the words of my mother's coworker, a fifty-year-old gym-goer: "Women are pigs."

I think men have this belief that should they find a secret peephole into their nearest women's locker room they would find lean, hard bodies sauntering about in various stages of undress, women's faces just barely obscured by rising clouds of steam. Gorgeous ladies talking and laughing, heads thrown back in outrageous slow-motion pleasure, long hair tossing to and fro. Some are naked; others are clad in lacy thongs and see-through bras, ever-so-gently massaging lotion into freshly shaven legs and, as the camera pans upward, a view of taut, tan abdomens. As the vision continues, naughty-looking babes at the vanity bend over to apply their makeup, their mouths parted in ecstasy as they line their lips in porn star cherry red.

Oh, if they only knew. Ready for a reality check? Here are some of the not-so-shy acts I have seen carried out before my very eyes: A woman sitting bareback on one of the maroon metal stools provided for members, one leg crossed at the knee, inspecting between her toes for, what—spare change? Grown women scrutinizing their pores just millimeters from the vertical fluorescent tubular lights that line the locker room's mirrors, popping their zits, and then proceeding un-fazed with their makeup routines. A woman, bent at the waist, taking a break from blow-drying her hair to, ummm, warm her nether regions, then continuing to style her hair as if a wholly unsanitary public act had not just occurred.

I once saw a woman pulling up the cellulite on her thighs and rear to see what they would look like if they were per-fectly smooth. Dream big, girlfriend! (Now, admit it: Many of us have done this before, but only in the privacy of our own bathrooms.)

Nancy, thirty-seven, had the unfortunate experience of be-ing initiated into the locker room by a woman who was blow-drying her hair in the buff, one leg up on the counter at *just* the right angle so that, with all the mirrors, "I could see her cervix and fallopian tubes." Talk about getting more than she'd bargained for; Nancy showed up for a shower and walked out a novice obstetrician/gynecologist.

A personal pet peeve: blood-stained tissues, used as make-shift shave accident bandages. Why do women let them fall to the ground and then leave them there? When I cut myself with one of the crappy razors provided by my gym (that is, before my petal pink epiphany), I tried to make sure the little square of tissue stuck. If it fell to the floor, I *picked it up.*

It's just as the kitschy plaques in those obnoxious, tchotchke-filled restaurant bathrooms say: "Your mother doesn't live here. Clean up after yourself." Don't leave your dirty, sopping-wet towels on the ground for the staff to pick up. Stop cleaning out your hairbrush and letting the tumbleweeds of hair float to the ground—I'll bet you a million dollars there's a wastebasket right around the corner. Stop peeing/blowing your nose in the shower, especially if someone's in the stall next to you. She doesn't want to stand in your body fluids as they flow by into the drain at the end of the shower bank. These little steps will make using the locker room infinitely more pleasurable, not to mention sanitary, for you and those around you.

Multiple Organisms

To get the dirt on all this dirt, I consulted Philip M. Tierno, Jr., PhD, Director of Clinical Microbiology and Immunology at New York University Medical Center and author of *The Secret Lives of Germs.* Considered in many circles the foremost authority on germs, Dr. Tierno is widely credited with unlocking the mystery between tampons and toxic shock syndrome. According to Tierno, germs in the locker room come from three sources: oral, skin, and fecal secretions. In addition to the germs we track in from our health club's dumbbells, sweaty bicycle seats, and ab mats, we also have to contend with other peoples' pathogenic germs, such as those that cause the flu, colds, and intestinal infections.

For protection, Dr. Tierno recommended some obvious tactics, such as always washing your hands before eating, drinking, and certainly after using the toilet. When it comes to walking barefoot in communal showers, slip on some flip-flops. This will help keep athlete's foot and warts at bay. Last, sitting nude on a stool provided by the locker room is not a good idea; you can pass all sorts of germs, from influenza to an infinitely icky-sounding disease he referred to as "crotch rot."

That's right. I said crotch rot.

So, I asked Dr. Tierno, is the locker room the germiest place a woman can be?

Not so. "The dirtiest place to be is the kitchen . . . especially the sink." Apparently sponges and dishrags can harbor everything from *E. coli 0157* to the genus *Salmonella enteritidis* and the genus *Shigella*.

If you remember nothing else, remember this, ladies. Listen to the good doctor. Stay out of the goddamn kitchen and order in! You owe it to your health!

7

Cellulite

The Bumpy Bane of My Existence

E very woman has cellulite. Period. If you don't, well, I'm sorry, but I just don't think we can be friends.

That's all.

8

A Steamy Situation
Talk, Sweat, and Tears in the Sauna

Wetness of unknown origin is a big issue for me. It freaks me out. If I'm wearing sandals and I step in a puddle and my toes get wet, I can easily spend the next three or four hours obsessing over the contents of that puddle: What bacteria and microorganisms were in it? Did anything sickly seep into me? Or, if I grab a railing on the bus and my thumb squishes along the metal into some gooey substance leftover by who knows what, my mind immediately runs through a catalog of bodily substances and associated pathogens that I may have come into contact with. Was it spit? Sweat? *Sperm*?! God forbid I sit on a damp bus seat. I might as well just hold the bus driver at knifepoint until he rushes me to the nearest emergency room to treat me for (a) gonorrhea, (b) a panic attack, or (c) some combination of the two.

So it seems counterintuitive that I would love the steam room so much. After all, when you think about it, what it is, essentially, is a hot box filled with other people's sweat; their perspiration emanates through their pores, slides off their bodies, and ultimately condenses. Then, it waits, droplets clinging desperately to the ceiling until the weight becomes too much to bear and they drip onto my forehead or into my cup of once-pure and refreshing ice water. Sick.

And yet, on a cold, blustery winter afternoon, as I leave work and head to the gym, all I can think about is my post-workout trip to the steam room. How good it will feel as I open the door and that steamy blast of air, 100-plus degrees, hits my face, instantly curling the hairs around my forehead and causing my eyes to squint as if I were fumbling in a dark room for the light switch. I search for a spot, careful not to sit down on some poor relaxing gal's face, and then . . . ahhhh. Sure, sometimes a woman will use the water hose to trigger the steam generator so that it gets too hot and my thighs end up looking like a Rorschach ink-blot test. Those are usually the days that, ten minutes after the shower, I'm *still* schvitzing and need to sit half-naked and read a magazine until my body releases the pent-up heat. But oh, is it worth it.

I love my time in the steam room because it is exactly that—my time. With one towel wrapped around my waist and one set out on the tiled bench, I stretch out and luxuriate in the hot mist. It envelops me as if it were my own private cloud, giving my mind time to wander from the most trivial of issues (which pajamas shall I wear tonight?) to the more serious matters taking up residence in my mind (will I ever want children?). Every so often, my train of thought is disrupted as the old pipes kick in and the steam starts up again. Like an orgasm, it begins with a few sputters of hot air, building to a crescendo-like string of stronger gusts, and finally, the climax, as the heat shoots out like an airy geyser, misting up the room again until I can hardly breathe.

Whew. Is it getting hot in here?

Hothouse Flower

Bizarre as it may sound, I was first introduced to the world of steam rooms and saunas by my grandfather, an avid runner and swimmer who also initiated what would turn out to be my lifelong pursuit of the perfect health club. At grandpa's gym, the dry sauna was coed and, following a long workout, we would meet, clad in our bathing suits and towels, where he would pour cups of water over the rocks and eucalyptus-filled steam would rise until all we had to go by was the sound of each other's voices.

When I was a teenager, I met a woman in that sauna, a beautiful black lady whose skin, flooded with rivulets of sweat, surely belied her age by many years. As we began talking, she revealed that she had been visiting the sauna for decades and believed she owed her nearly flawless skin (she was in her early sixties with nary a wrinkle) to, more than anything, the heat. The steam. The sweat.

Ever since my teens, I've been hooked on steam rooms—not searching-between-your-toes-for-a-vein hooked, but more like really-needing-a-hard-drink-right-now hooked. The sauna gets me hot for a number of reasons, among them what I believe to be its many health benefits, such as meditation, reduced muscle stiffness, and some damn potent, herbal-enhanced sinus clearing. You also always hear people talk about "sweating out toxins" in the steam room, but I wondered whether that might be an urban myth, like the one about gum and how it takes seven years to pass through you or the belief that Pop Rocks and Coca-Cola explode in your stomach. So I sought out an expert, Elizabeth Tanzi, MD, a clinical instructor of dermatology at the Johns Hopkins University School of Medicine and the codirector of the

Washington Institute of Dermatologic Laser Surgery in Washington, D.C.

Indeed, Dr. Tanzi said there is no scientific proof that one can literally sweat out toxins. But she did agree that the steam room can open up pores and ease aches and pains. The warm, soothing nature relaxes us, she said. "That's why it feels so good." Sensitive-skinned patients should avoid the heat, but, Dr. Tanzi said, the steam room can be quite a hydrating experience, especially when followed with a shower and ample moisturizer.

But far more than the hot-air-and-a-lube job, I love the steam room for the meaning I have always instilled in it. Watching television as a child, I found the images of women in saunas with their hair wrapped turban-style helped shape my perception of what it meant to be a *woman*—no girls allowed. This was the place ladies gathered to dish about sex, love, their bodies, *men*'s bodies. Women and their steam rooms were like men and their cigar bars, bachelors and their strip clubs, mobsters and their backdoor gambling rooms. It was a club I wanted to be a part of—a room of one's own. Now that I am old enough, I savor the days when I have an extra fifteen minutes to spread out a towel and just sweat my cares away. (Or, as the case may be, to stew in my own angry juices.) Whether it's completely empty or I have to fight for a spot, I can never resist the steam room's siren call.

See Jill Sweat. See Jill Chat.
Should Jill Shut Up?

I often prefer silence in the steam room. It offers me a chance to be still, to take in the day's events and plan tomorrow's, as if that's possible. Unfortunately, sometimes the silence is punctured by an odd moan of relaxation. These boudoir sighs I do not understand. I'm feeling just as unwound as these other women are, but you don't hear me heaving and exhaling the way Jenna Jameson does, do you?

"Mmmmm," I hear from across the room (and it's not a big room), noticing faint movement as she takes a big gulp of water and shifts from left butt cheek to right.

"Ughhhh," as another wipes her face and places her feet up on the wall at a ninety-degree angle, knees at least twelve inches apart. Am I being filmed? Because I'm half-naked and I'd best be receiving royalties.

Better is the girl talk; this kind of noise I don't mind one bit. Steam-room chitchat is the greatest. This is hot gossip— literally. I've discovered fabulous sushi restaurants, heard tales of horrendous break-ups, and learned where to go for the best shoe bargains in the city, just by lying back and listening to girls gab in the steam room. Other women may find this annoying, but for me, if I'm in the right mood, it can be as satisfying as reading a juicy entertainment magazine or watching mindless television.

For my friend Diane, twenty-eight, however, when it comes to the steam room, the quieter, the better. Sure, she's heard the occasional moan or groan, which, admittedly, is a bit awkward; but, as she considerately put it, to each her own. However, Diane is annoyed by women who walk in and proceed to launch into loud, obnoxious conversations. When one views the steam room as a quiet area, she said, loud talk is "disrespectful to the space."

I suppose I can see both sides. For some, the steam room is a silent sanctuary, a place to escape with your thoughts, and yours alone. For others, it's a place to socialize. Myself, I swing both ways. I even met two new friends at my gym by semi-eavesdropping on their steam-room banter. It seemed Vicki, thirty-six, and Eleanor, fifty-nine, were joined at the hip, always chatting away and *always* doing so in the steam room. What they talked about, I'm not really sure; I didn't listen that closely as I lay on my towel in the foggy heat. It was more of a white noise type of thing, but I could tell by the tone and rapidity of their voices that they were having fun. And I wanted in on it. So I made it a point to introduce myself to them one day, after my steam and shower.

Vicki, who has been steaming for a decade or so, used to spend time in the dry sauna. But before long she was yearning for something hotter, so she slipped next door, tried the wet steam, and was instantly hooked. She finds it cathartic and makes it a point to join Eleanor every Friday morning for at least five minutes, no matter how busy the two of them are. "It's a bonding experience," Vicki described, echoing my previous childhood sentiments of seeing images of women in the steam room and equating that with adult friendships and sacred connections. After she and Eleanor met and clicked, they found the steam room was the perfect conduit for gabbing about everything from relationships to work, family, recipes, weekend plans and—golden rule be damned—other people.

But don't get her wrong—Vicki's not always chitchatting in the steam room. When alone, she uses it as an escape, an opportunity to flex her emotional muscles while relaxing her physical ones. Sometimes a simple fifteen minutes of sweltering solitude is enough to help her channel her creativity as she plans her next meal, her next workday, her next writing assignment.

Amiee, thirty-three, has had many open and amusing conversations in the sauna, typically with complete strangers. Her hypothesis: A small, intimate setting such as a sauna or steam room makes some people more inclined to open up. For example, the woman who started asking Amiee about her dating life soon revealed that she had fallen in love over the Internet with a personal trainer in Florida. They'd been "dating" for months but had not yet met face-to-face. Or another woman who, around Christmas, struck up a friendly conversation about all the things she had purchased. She asked where Amiee shopped, what gifts she had bought, and more, but the stranger then proceeded to talk about how much her husband hates it when she spends money and about all of the financial debt she'd gotten them into over the years. "I was friendly, but I didn't ask for these details!" Amiee exclaimed.

The best are the women (yes, plural) whom Amiee has seen/heard talking on cell phones in the sauna. I can just picture it: "Can you hear me now?" (Lies down, feet up.) "Can you hear me now?" (Sits up, readjusts towel turban.) "Can you hear me now? Good."

Eleanor, Vicki's steam mate, has been hitting the heat for three decades (which may explain her smooth-as-a-baby's-Botoxed-bottom skin), and it all started with a Turkish bath house here in Chicago, which has now been converted into a chi-chi Asian restaurant. Thirty years ago, the sauna was for males only, except for Wednesday evenings, when women of all ages would flock to the grand, column-fronted building for "Ladies' Night." There, Eleanor would linger for up to four hours with her girlfriends, hopping from the dry sauna to the whirlpools, then into the steam room, where they would whip one another with huge palm fronds to stimulate circulation. They would eat and drink (as in, alcohol), play games; sometimes they would henna their hair, even though that was against the rules. Women would dump buckets of cold water over each other's heads to cool down; others would "throw," meaning throw water on the rocks in the dry sauna to produce more steam. The whole experience, as Eleanor described it, was extremely social.

"You'd be laughing and throwing water. Sometimes the Gypsies would come and steal your shampoo!"

Today, Eleanor steams in our locker room at least once a week. Sometimes she'll stay in as long as she can stand it and then just go home and pass out—not literally, but I know what she means. After twenty minutes in the steam room, it's often all I can do to get dressed and into my car because I am just so damned relaxed I feel almost narcoleptic. I believe I've even slipped into the lightest phase of sleep while in the steam room, just from the cozy tranquility of it all. (Oy, I can hear my mother freaking out right now.)

Popping My Friend's Steam Room Cherry

I had the privilege of introducing my dear friend Diane to the steam room a few years ago at my health club. With her wild, curly dark brown hair and a small touch of claustrophobia, she had never really considered it, for trichological as well as psychological reasons. But as it is with so many firsts in life (your first Dragon roll, your first leap out of an airplane, buying your first dildo), it helps to have a girlfriend there. So in we went, towels wrapped 'round our chests, sitting side by side and taking a steam.

She loved it.

Her last gym had a great steam room, and she began to use it about three times a week for fifteen minutes at a go, or as long as she could stand it. "I love that feeling of just sweating," Diane said. "For me, a good workout means sweating. That, to me, means I've worked my body hard, I'm keeping myself in shape. And in the steam room, it feels cleansing. It feels like you're doing something good for yourself. You kind of get addicted to it."

As her experience in the steam room has grown, so has her comfort level with nudity. At first, she used three towels: one wrapped around her hair, one around her body, and one to lie down on. But as she's grown more at ease with her surroundings, she's come to recognize that steam roomies aren't there to judge. Nobody cares, and besides, who can see through all that steam?

"There's large, small, skinny, fat. You realize nobody's looking at you and you're like, 'Screw it! Why am I leaving early because I'm uncomfortably hot when I could stay later and just take my towel off?'" So she'll take it off and maybe lay it across her lap, napkin-like, for propriety's sake.

As for me, I've experimented with everything from just topless to the whole shebang, and I have to say that I prefer the former, if for nothing more than safety's sake. Little Leslie from Down Below isn't designed to be exposed to harsh elements like extreme heat, especially in her newly nude state, so coverage of some sort is a necessity.

One thing I will say is that, much like wearing all black or having a nice faux tan, glistening with steam-room sweat does wonders for a woman's body. You instantly look slimmer, your muscles are highlighted in all the right places . . . you just look sexy. At least that's how I feel. I tend to lie with my arms crossed at my chest, and the other day I looked down (for research purposes, of course) and, I must say, my boobs looked *fantastic,* glossy with sweat and framed like a mountain relief by my biceps and forearms. Maybe if geography was this much fun in school I would actually know where the Dakotas are today!

Achtung, Baby!

Amiee, the woman who feels as if she were starring in a commercial for cell phones every time she steams, grew up in Germany, where saunas abound. If a town has the word *Bad* in it, as in *Bad* Kitzingen or *Bad* Orb, it means there is a sauna or spa there. In Germany, and throughout Europe, it is fairly standard practice for any athlete to proceed directly to the showers and then to the sauna after an athletic game or practice. It usually starts young, around twelve or thirteen, said Amiee, who played soccer throughout high school. The sauna was a place to recoup after games and stretch out sore muscles—coaches' orders. Sometimes talking was not even allowed. But that was their sauna culture, and it was ingrained in her lifestyle. So when she moved to the United States and started scouting out health clubs, a good, proper sauna was at the top of her list.

But there is something about American saunas that leaves Amiee steamed: the patrons. More specifically, their behavior. Back in Germany, one would never enter without having showered after a workout, whereas we dirty Americans go straight from Stairmaster to steam room. I'll be the first to admit it, I do. It had never even occurred to me to shower before sweating; the same reasoning I use when I leave my bed unmade in the morning because hey, I'm just going to rumple the comforter up again that night.

Unfortunately, Amiee has seen worse than straight-to-sauna sauntering; things that would gross me out, too, like women lying down while still in their sweaty workout gear . . . shoes included! I agree with her when she labels such behavior disgusting. Sometimes women will place their clean clothes in her sauna while they shower so they have a toasty outfit to change into when they're finished. Although it's not the most sanitary of practices, in the dead of winter, I find this idea rather inspired. But still. Ew. You can't trust strangers' cleanliness.

She partly attributes the bizarre behavior to her gym's inexplicable "No Nudity" policy for the wooden hot box. Excuse me, but no nudity in the sauna?! No nudity is more oppressive a rule than people my height having to fly coach. It sounds not only extremely uncomfortable but borderline torturous. As Amiee pointed out, one of the main purposes of a sauna is to open your pores and release the gunk. How can you do that with Spinning shorts and a tank clinging to your skin? She's not suggesting that anyone enter without a towel—she always places one wherever her body touches the wood—but as for clothes and shoes, nuh-uh. Amiee goes nude, even if the sign says not to, because, well, "I think those rules are stupid." Go on with your *Bad* self, Amiee!

Amiee isn't the only one to have caught the sauna bug while abroad. Catherine, forty-three, has sweated it out in Budapest, Iceland, and a host of Scandinavian countries, and now she uses the sauna about six times per week. She's worked her way up to about twenty-five minutes per session and loves every naked, muscle-relaxing, uninhibited minute of it.

Catherine loves both the meditative and social aspects of the sauna. The latter came into play more when she was traveling abroad, she said, and she added, "There are more saunas in Finland than cars." Her helpful analogy: "What pubs are to the Irish, saunas are to the Icelandic."

She described those international saunas (and accompanying "pools" into which you dip before and after a session in the sauna) as liberating in that, no matter what your body type, you were free to pop in and out, without judgment of being too this or too that. Note: There is no "fat" in Finland, no "butt" in Budapest. In fact, in Budapest, where bathhouses abound, Catherine said, body image rarely enters your mind when you're surrounded by "very heavy Eastern European women. They don't care." So why should we?

Regarding the meditative aspect, Catherine said she appreciates the fact that when she emerges from our hometown sauna six days a week, she can always count on feeling more in touch with her body and mind. Just like a vacation that takes years off one's stressed-out face, the sauna is a sped-up massage, a holiday-in-a-capsule. "There are no men there," she said, "no competition. You just sit. And. Relax."

9

Throwing Our Weight Around
Plus-Sized in the Land of Thin

*I felt like I got watched, like women would
watch me get undressed to feel better about themselves.
So I'd change in the bathroom stalls.*—Jennifer

*When you're morbidly obese, you can see people
looking at you out of the corner of their eye,
or the subtle nudge to a friend.*—Annie

*You know what's worse than the glares, the stares,
the one-liners? The total isolation. No wonder America
continues to sit on the couch and get bigger and bigger.
It's the last and greatest remaining discrimination.
We're merciless.*—Dee

Right Under My Nose

It's ironic that Dee, above, spoke to me of isolation, of being
ignored by the "skinny minnies" who surround her at health
clubs and in locker rooms. For when I made my inaugural

visit to a local meeting of a national chain weight-loss support group, I was surprised to find it was located in a spot I've passed hundreds of times before. I must have walked by the storefront, in a small strip mall situated across from my neighborhood coffeehouse, daily at times, simply failing to notice the bold red letters announcing the business being conducted inside. I couldn't help but wonder: Does this render me as guilty as the skinny minnies who foster a sense of seclusion in the overweight women in my locker room?

At the front desk, an older woman greeted me warmly and asked whether she could help me. I told her I was interested in sitting in on a session. She asked my name and neatly wrote it on a sticky badge, along with the word "Visitor" in bold letters underneath. I certainly don't think she meant to, but by doing so, she made me feel like an outsider, as if I didn't belong. Those seven letters announced to the room that I was simply stopping by and soon enough I'd be on my merry way. I slapped the sticker on my chest and entered the stockroom-style meeting area.

Inside, I found women of all shapes and sizes—in fact, more seemed to be healthy than obese—donning everything from pastel tweed suits to athletic gear to leopard print skirts and matching pumps. Two men rounded out the group (one, a dead ringer for Steve Buscemi). Everyone carried a bottle of water or a steaming cup of coffee as if it were an extra appendage. At the far end of the room was a private weighing area; from here people emerged clutching passport-like pamphlets, their weights stamped inside like foreign locales. Only instead of "Italy," "South Africa," and "Aruba," their documents read "175 pounds, Feb. 5, 2005" or "172.5 pounds, Feb. 12, 2005." Destinations of a different sort.

I had come to gather some insight into the mind-set of the heavyset, but most people there looked only mildly over-weight. One exercise initiated by the freakishly smiley and very thin group leader, however, did turn up some interesting remarks. The man in charge, who had recently lost nearly 100 pounds, asked people to generate a list of "feeling words" to describe how they felt when they saw a photo of themselves that just didn't jibe with how they pictured themselves. A body image project—jackpot! He flipped over a fresh sheet of poster paper and started writing. Some of the words that people shouted out:

Disgust
Embarrassment
Sadness
Disappointment
Anxiety
Anger

The Other Side

Despite the wishful thinking of men—and, I suppose, women—everywhere, the ladies' locker room is not filled with only young, lithe women, rosy-faced from Spin class and racing to meet their girlfriends for cosmos and California rolls. There is a much-ignored segment that deserves atten-tion, too: plus-sized women. Whether they are avidly trying to lose weight or are happy just the way they are, overweight women lift the same dumbbells, use the same saunas, and face the same body-image woes as everyone else.

In her book *Fat Girls and Lawn Chairs,* Cheryl Peck opens with a true-to-life health-club vignette that goes something like this: Peck, weighing in at approximately 300 pounds but nonetheless working it out at the gym, is sitting on a bench in the locker room. She is half naked. She is minding her own business. That's when a fellow exerciser, about twenty years younger with a taut little body and sexy, support-free undergarments, leans over to Peck and says, "I just wanted to tell you—I admire you for coming here every day. You give me inspiration to keep coming myself."

Hmmm. I imagine if I were Peck, such a comment would make me wonder, "Gee, thanks. Now what the fuck is that supposed to mean?"

So I called Peck and asked her myself. And indeed, she said that although the exchange, which she labeled the "inspirational goddess" incident, made her think, "You've got to be kidding me," it also left her wondering what, exactly, the compliment was. Although she's fairly confident the young woman meant no harm, for Peck, it came across as backhanded and condescending. She didn't need to be anyone's inspirational—or thinspirational, while we're at it—goddess. She was simply trying to get in shape because her girlfriend wanted the two of them to walk the Appalachian Trail together and Peck was nowhere near ready. Besides that, she was starting to get hooked on the whole exercise-induced endorphin rush thing.

Despite the title of her book, Peck refers to herself as "a person of size." She admitted that it is difficult for people of size to accept a compliment about their bodies because "they're so rare." On the flip side, the ones doing the flattering sometimes aren't very graceful, simply because they don't know how to do it properly.

Ch-ch-ch-changing

Brooke, twenty-nine, is five foot one and weighs 200 pounds. She gained most of the extra weight in college, largely a result of smoking too much pot and then succumbing to too many Cool Ranch Doritos. Now, she belongs to a gym as well as a studio specializing in personal training. Brooke eats healthfully but still, in spite of all of this, she cannot shed the weight.

She doesn't change in her locker room, mostly because she lives right across the street. However, she confessed, her dressing habits are partly influenced by the fact that there are "a billion skinny girls walking around, talking, doing their makeup." Brooke would never change in front of them. In fact, just the other day, she witnessed two thin young women callously whispering about a third girl who, although a bit on the plump side, most people would not have considered overweight. It's that type of unforgiving atmosphere that prevents Brooke from taking advantage of the privileges she could enjoy in the locker room, such as taking trips to the sauna (where half of the towels don't fit).

This sense of isolation has caused Dee, forty-eight, to change clubs. And who can blame her, when she explained: "Can you imagine—you don't even get a smile, you don't get a 'Hello'? That's worse than being called a name." She's seen some overweight women change in the shower stall, so afraid are they of being stared at or teased. Much the way young children learn not to touch the hot stove, these women have learned the lesson: If something is going to hurt, avoid it.

Jennifer is one of those women who changes in the bathroom stalls. At five foot six and 240 pounds, Jennifer is clinically obese, and yet she fences four nights a week, for up to four hours per session. The thirty-two-year-old is not interested in losing weight—she subscribes to the fat-but-fit theory—but detests the stares and glares she receives in the locker room because they seem to drip with pity: "Oh, poor thing has to work out."

The wonderful irony, however, is that Jennifer could "kick most of these girls' butts." I don't doubt her—the woman can leg-press 500 pounds. Yet despite the strong exterior shell, underneath the layers of muscle and, yes, fat, lays a vulnerable interior. As she gets undressed, she can't help but feel that other women watch her, hawk-like, in a deplorable attempt to feel better about themselves. To deny them such sadistic privilege, she'll change in the bathroom stalls. Especially if the women voyeurs are the types who apply makeup *before* they work out. Such vanity is proof positive for Jennifer that it's time to hit the toilets to get undressed. Better to change where people shit then where people are shitty, I suppose.

I wish Jennifer had been around to kick my butt when I experienced what I consider one of my most judgmental moments in the locker room. It was the dead of winter and I was changing next to a very large woman. As she struggled to get her boots off, then her jacket and pants, huffing and puffing all the while, I couldn't control the tiny twinge I felt of . . . not pity, but I guess what you could call unasked-for empathy. A bright, beet-red hue was spreading across her face and, at precisely the wrong moment, she caught me staring. Eye to eye. I desperately wanted to crawl into my locker and have someone throw away the combination. Who was I, someone who had struggled on and off for years with an eating disorder, to pass judgment on another woman with an eating issue of another kind?

And then, the slap to the face.

The woman opened her mouth and I steeled myself for a well-deserved dressing-down. But she said, with a softened expression, "Just you wait until you're eight months pregnant . . . "

Ugh.

". . . and your asthma starts acting up."

Double ugh.

I smiled weakly, but felt so, so ashamed inside. I still do.

Turning a Negative into a Positive

As it turned out, not all plus-sized women I spoke with have had negative experiences in the locker room. Take Krista, who is thirty-two, for example. Krista's not overweight now, but she used to be. Although even she recognizes that at her heaviest—five foot and 155 pounds—she was not exactly obese (in fact, wearing a size 14, she fit the national average), she was not at a healthy weight, either. But being overweight was not a deterrent for her when it came to the locker room. In truth, Krista said, she found the environment a positive, liberating opportunity to witness the reality of women's bodies.

"You can see stretch marks, rolls, tattoos," she described. And she's right: Even women who look the best in their running shorts and T-back fitted tanks reveal imperfections when fluorescent lighting shines on their nakedness. Abandoned by Spandex and washed free of concealer, we are all flawed: For Krista, that was comforting—a sort of great equalizer that helped her worldview morph from fantasy to reality.

Periodic workouts at a nearby university gym also proved especially helpful in overcoming anxiety about her weight.

Here, she found, even the most elite varsity competitors had the occasional saggy bits. And even though they were just that—bits—they were enough to embolden her to disrobe, minus the pity party.

Not that it's much of an issue for her anymore. Thanks to that tried-and-true combination of eating well, regular exercise, and a long-term commitment to an active, healthy lifestyle, Krista now fluctuates between a healthy size 4 and 6. She is a personal trainer and runs a Web site dedicated to weight training. She fought her pounds and won.

Krista has friends who have admitted to being jealous of her figure, which disturbs her, particularly because she doesn't believe there was anything special about the way she went about losing her weight, a method she refers to as "democratic." She confessed there is still a part of her inside that feels overweight, though, that carries the burden of being an overweight woman. It's not that she feels there is anything wrong with her, she explained, but rather that her mind retains an internally processed image of herself at her previous size. Sometimes she'll pick out the wrong article of clothing when shopping, instinctively grabbing for the size 14 rather than the size 4, and she believes that if she drew a picture of herself, or picked a size that she believed was hers, the result would probably look heavier than her actual image.

In the locker room, Krista has made it over to the other side of the proverbial fence. She feels that she now blends in more easily—perhaps the ultimate goal for women of all sizes who simply want to get in and out of their gym clothes (but maybe look just a little bit hot in between). Her reduced frame may bear fewer pounds, but it is stronger from carrying a heavier amount of confidence. In addition to that, Krista now feels she has the luxury of no longer caring what others think of her . . . although she is aware that people now treat her as "one of those mythical, naturally skinny people," which bothers her a bit. "Thin," she said, is not an adjective for which she strives. "Actually the idea of being 'thin' kind of grosses me out because I equate it with being weak and frail." If she could maintain the same level of body fat and put on 20 pounds of muscle, she'd do it in an instant.

My Enormous Ass

Many women battling their own weight-loss woes turn to blogs to post their progress and gain support from other women in the same situation. One woman in particular, Kristy, thirty, caught my eye with a ridiculously amusing, true-life story that described her being caught in a compromising position at her gym. I retell it here, for I feel stories like these need to be passed down so that our granddaughters, should they one day find themselves struggling with body image, can look back, laugh, and say, "At least Grammy once won an award for that story she wrote, 'Why Yes, Cute Fireman, That IS My Ass.'"

Kristy, who has always been conscious of her weight and recently was on a mission to shed the pounds she had gained after her divorce, was doing some circuit training at her gym. She was working out on a certain machine that works your hamstrings and glutes by placing you in a modified, all-fours position. You then kick back on a weighted pedal like a donkey, causing your butt to feel, shall we say, *en fuego*.

In the middle of her donkey-kick exercise, fire trucks began to pull up outside. But, being a city girl used to hearing bells and whistles at all hours of the night, Kristy kept on kicking. After all, it wasn't as if her gym was on fire. (As it turned out, the trucks were responding to reports of fumes nearby.) But I suspect that what propelled her story to on-line fame was the fact that as she was grunting and kicking away, she eventually came to the horrifying realization that, and I quote, "a SECRET and SILENT truck had pulled up DIRECTLY outside the window that was DIRECTLY behind the machine and so about a half-dozen firemen were parked in a way as to be DIRECTLY FACING MY ASS." Kristy supplemented this account with a hysterical, meticulously detailed mathematical diagram, showing a stick-figure drawing of her on the machine and two flesh colored balloons standing in for what she labeled "My enormous ass."

Kristy has since recovered from the incident, at least enough to talk in depth about her experiences in the locker room. Her first experience in an adult locker room was in college, when she decided to lose weight and get into great physical shape. Although not overweight as a child, she recently found a diary entry from when she was seven years old that read, "My tummy is bigger than other girls' tummies." Funny how distorted our perceptions can be—and at such an early age. In her college locker room, she still changed in the bathroom stall, for two reasons: If she saw that someone's body was "better" than hers, she felt ugly; and if she saw another woman with stretch marks or who was overweight, she feared that was what she looked like to other people. Changing in the open was simply a lose-lose situation.

Now, Kristy is far less self-conscious about her body, but still considers herself hyper-aware. Regardless, she insists on maintaining a good sense of humor about her weight, as evidenced by the fire-truck story. As she put it, "Whatever

I'm walking around with is the best I've got at that particular time."

A Stitch in Their Sides

For a growing number of women, however, whatever they're walking around with is not only *not* the best they've got, it's downright dangerous. For them, baby fat has grown into chunkiness, then into overweight, and eventually into obesity. According to the National Center for Health Statistics, part of the Centers for Disease Control and Prevention (CDC), approximately 65 percent of Americans aged twenty or older are either overweight or obese. During the past two decades, obesity has dramatically increased in the United States. In fact, in 2005, the CDC estimated that obesity ranked number seven among the nation's leading causes of preventable death.

"Obesity in general is one of the most potent predictors of diabetes, heart disease, depression, sleep apnea, osteoporosis—it's on a causal pathway to just about all of the leading causes of disease in our society," said David L. Katz, MD, MPH, director of Yale University School of Medicine's Prevention Research Center and one of the nation's leading experts on obesity. With such obvious links, no one needs to be spoon-fed the obvious: Being overweight is dangerous, even deadly.

Psychologically speaking, Dr. Katz has seen the devastating effects that a preoccupation with being overweight can have on a woman's self-esteem. A person may be intelligent, interesting, involved in numerous social activities, loved by many people, but when she characterizes herself in words, she always mentions the word *fat*: "Excess adipose tissue becomes the dominant trait they see in themselves," said Dr. Katz. He tries to help his patients unbundle their weight from their personalities so that they can see themselves as people worthy of more than just that one unforgiving adjective.

Many people, for whom diet and exercise have just not worked, have found an answer in gastric bypass, a surgery that makes the stomach smaller and allows food to bypass part of the small intestine. Patients feel full more quickly, which reduces the amount of food taken in, and, thus, calories consumed. In addition, bypassing part of the intestine results in decreased calorie absorption. *Et voilà*—the pounds melt away.

According to the American Society for Bariatric Surgery (ASBS) (which encompasses gastric bypass), at least 171,000 patients underwent some type of bariatric surgery in 2005. That's up from 36,700 in the year 2000—a *366 percent increase*. Even more astounding, those figures, they say, are most likely major underestimates, because they take into account only physicians who are members of the ASBS—many doctors performing the procedures are not, and therefore they do not report them to the society.

One of the most open advocates for gastric bypass has been the singer Carnie Wilson, most recognized for her years in the musical trio Wilson Phillips and as the daughter of Brian Wilson of the Beach Boys. After a lifetime struggle with her weight, Wilson opted for the surgery when her scale hit 300 pounds (although she believes she weighed more—the scale simply didn't register higher). At that point, body image wasn't at the top of her list of priorities; health was.

"Body image is one thing, morbid obesity is terrifying," Wilson divulged during our phone conversation as she nursed her newborn baby, Lola Sophia. "I was going to die. It wasn't just looking good and being toned. I had sleep apnea and high blood pressure and was pre-diabetic and had slipped disks in my back. My feet hurt [from carrying the excess weight]."

Wilson's 1999 gastric bypass was televised on the Internet, like the Victoria's Secret annual fashion show. After the procedure, she eventually dropped to 146 pounds, leveling out at a stable 150. But the descent from a size 28 to a size 6 did not bring her instant comfort with her body. For instance, Wilson said that at her heaviest weight, the only times she entered a locker room environment would be at a spa, and at those moments she was "embarrassed of the rolls of fat." But when she shed the pounds—the equivalent of an entire person—the locker room remained a stressful space because she was self-conscious of the excess skin and the scars from the reconstructive and plastic surgery she had to tighten it up (including a tummy tuck and breast lift). No matter whether she was in front of her mother, her sisters, or strangers, she felt ashamed.

Stretch marks remained a locker room worry for Wilson as well. An early developer, Wilson had stretch marks dating back to the fourth grade, and had accumulated even more through her weight gain and rapid weight loss. So the taste of success was especially sweet when, at her photo shoot for *Playboy* shortly after her weight loss, she looked up to see a giant unretouched picture of Anna Nicole Smith (taken right when she was discovered) that showed her "tons of stretch marks." I bring this up not to hate on Anna Nicole, but to show that everyone—*Playboy* bunnies included—has flaws. Nobody is immune. And Wilson's naughty side continues to come out when, if she is forced into a locker room (she avoids them at all costs . . . wouldn't you if you had a full gym at home with A/C, cable TV, plants, and hand-picked artwork on the wall?) she hides behind her robe and just looks. She admitted, like so many of us, "What I love is when I see a younger woman with a stretch mark."

(Ladies, this is called schadenfreude—it's that guilty little feeling of glee that takes over when a friend or other individual in your position fails. In the locker room, schadenfreude is your best friend. Embrace her and she will bring you much inner peace.)

For now, Wilson, thirty-eight, is focusing on balancing her baby, marriage, career—she recently recorded a solo album titled, appropriately, "Lolabies"—and getting her weight back on track. She gained 70 pounds during her pregnancy, reaching a high of 240, so she's been walking on the treadmill or outside in nature to help shed the weight. The endorphins make her feel on top of the world, as if she could conquer anything. A trainer guides her through Pilates, weight training, and yoga as well. There are still some procedures she wouldn't mind having—lifts for the butt, thighs, and chin come to mind—but she balances the body stuff out with the fact that she's "a good person and my husband loves me." She speaks out at hospitals and health expos on gastric bypass. And she encourages women, no matter what their weight or size, to celebrate the parts of their bodies that they do like, even if it means their hands or their hair. When you appreciate and take care of yourself, she believes, you feel better about your body. For instance, Wilson has always treated herself to salt scrubs, pedicures, and massages. She is not shy to admit that she's always had soft skin and smelled good. "It's amazing what a ten-dollar pedicure will do towards boosting your self-esteem and your femininity," she said. "It makes you feel delicious and like a woman at any size."

This, I believe, is fantastic advice and I'm totally set to jump in the tub with my new vanilla-coconut sugar scrub. But in all truthfulness, I'd rather have a life-sized, unretouched photo of a *Playboy* model to whip out, just in case I'm having a bad body-image day. Nothing says "Buck up, Little Camper," like a tushy zit on a bleached-blonde bunny.

Other women I spoke with who had undergone weight-loss surgery cited reasons similar to Wilson's, such as severe heath problems and a very real fear of dying. I talked with Brandi, thirty, just a shade over a week after her gastric by-pass surgery. She had already lost 15 pounds. Overweight since grade school, Brandi recalled starting on Richard Simmons's Deal-a-Meal program when she was ten, then moving to diet pills when that didn't work. She decided on bariatric surgery for a number of reasons, including the fact that her paternal grandmother died very young and obese and she desperately did not want to follow suit. At five foot seven and 323 pounds, Brandi longed for the chance to shop at trendy stores such as the Gap, to be unafraid of breaking rides at amusement parks, to sit comfortably in airplane seats, and to observe cute or thin girls without quietly murmuring such compliments as "Bitch" or "Slut."

Brandi has avoided locker rooms all her life because they make her feel too self-conscious. Unlike the svelte gym gals sauntering about in cute, tiny underwear, she has just never felt comfortable in the space. Perhaps that might change during the next twelve to eighteen months as she lunches daily on four bites of cottage cheese and two sips of apple juice on her way toward her goal of 175 pounds.

But a surprise threw Brandi for a loop just weeks after her surgery: She was pregnant. Tests confirmed that she was three weeks along during the operation. Her doctor doesn't seem to be concerned, but I can't help but wonder how this baby is going to thrive on a few sips of juice a day. Did the general anesthesia affect the fetus? How about the fact that Brandi's hair is falling out because of the lack of protein in her diet, and her skin is dry and flaky?

So far, Brandi has lost "only" 43 pounds since her surgery two months ago and has not joined a gym as planned. Not only has she been very ill with morning sickness, but, like Wilson, she now finds herself embarrassed not just about being heavy but also about her scars.

"I think about [undressing in the locker room], but then I remember my scars, my huge square butt, the cottage cheese on my huge square butt, and I just can't," she lamented. "I see other women much bigger in the locker room and I am happy I had the surgery and in some ways I want to show off, but nobody there knows I have a reason to be proud of my body, that it is shrinking. I don't want to be another fat chick in the locker room; I want to be the one they all look at and say, 'Wow, she is beautiful!' I know I won't ever have a bikini body. I just want to be something special. Chubby [is] fine with me . . . so long as I am not an ugly fat chick anymore. But at the moment, I still am. Someday, I will hit the locker room and change in front of everyone there. I would consider myself having 'made it' when I can get to that point."

Brandi's comments brought tears to my eyes. No mother-to-be who has just gone through a life-changing surgery should think of herself as an "ugly fat chick." No mother-to-be should visit other girls' online pregnancy boards and see pictures of skinny women with cute little bumps and cry because she "may never look pregnant." Apparently surgery isn't the cure-all many of us thought it to be.

Annie, forty-two, opted for an operation even more radical than traditional gastric bypass. Called the duodenal switch, it removed the majority of her stomach, allowing food to bypass 80 percent of her intestines. She lost 200 pounds. Size 30 to size 4. From 335 pounds to 135. Damn.

The surgery left her with a railroad-like incision from below her bra-line to her belly button, held together by staple after staple. And as her body rapidly shed the excess pounds, her skin lost its elasticity, leaving her once plumped-up body like a deflated balloon. Like Wilson, she wound up having multiple surgeries to remove excess skin, including a tummy tuck that took off 5 pounds.

So Annie's body image went on quite a roller coaster ride, as one might expect—especially in the locker room. Prior to "the Switch," Annie would go to great lengths to avoid any display of the skin, so afraid was she of being stared at or ridiculed. Even though nobody would actually go so far as to make a comment in the locker room, she would definitely hear an occasional "Tsk" of disapproval or even shock, or an under-the-breath "Oh my God." Eventually, the stage-whispered harassment simply stopped her from going to the gym.

But then, after taking time off from work after her surgery to speed the weight loss, Annie found her body image still under attack. She would work out only at low-traffic times because the torsal scar served as an ever-present reminder of what she wasn't able to do on her own: "I had to go and get someone to change my entire digestive tract," she said. But at the same time, there was no denying that the surgery had worked. Once Annie was able to stop looking at the scar as a symbol of failure and as just another part of her body, she was okay. And the locker room became a safe place for her.

Phat Camp

I knew Marilyn Wann was somebody I wanted to get to know better when, responding to my email, she signed off, "Marilyn Wann, Author/Troublemaker." A leading fat activist who wrote the book *Fat!So?* and proudly refers to herself as "flabulous," Wann weighs 270 pounds, has a personal trainer, and works out three times a week, doing yoga, lifting weights, swimming, and walking. Her doctor, she said, has told her she's healthy, that all the necessary numbers are in the normal range.

Unlike so many overweight women, Wann described the locker room as being "home" to her. She doesn't go there assuming something bad is going to happen, that a rude gesture will ruin her workout or a hurtful remark will mar her mind-set. In fact, she enjoys her unapologetic attitude, and often makes it a point to "put herself in the faces" of these people who view the soft, round parts of the body as things to be removed or burned away through running, sweating, liposuction.

"I'm not hiding, scuttering around," Wann said. "I'm just there, doing my thing like anyone else doing their thing. It's kind of fun to perform the self-celebrating, self-accepting fat person identity in that space."

Sometimes Wann will find herself chatting in the locker room with other women from the fat acceptance community and she'll notice people listening in on their conversation, simply because it's so different from what they're used to talking about. Because she often hangs out with other fat activists, they may be talking about "things that have horrified us, like that Kirstie Alley is a big fat sell out [for pimping for Jenny

Craig so soon after her show, *Fat Actress,* hit the air], or how the CDC just came out with revised obesity rates . . . or how good it feels to work out. But we never talk about what we weigh or what we've been eating." In fact, when Wann sees thin women step onto the scale, only to descend with saddened, distraught looks on their faces, it is she who feels sad for them. Meanwhile, she—all 270 pounds of her—is being noisy and happy and "taking up space on the little bench."

"Fat liberation is really just common sense," she explained. "We've gotten so twisted around by the marketing of 'Be thin, be thin.' My common sense says nobody's life needs to be determined by the number on the bathroom scale." Wann shuns the notion that one shouldn't go to the gym unless one is already in shape. This, she feels, is analogous to many women's belief that they must tidy up the house before the cleaning service comes. Wann also avoids the use of the adjective "plus-sized" because "then what are thin people— 'minus-sized'?" Her bottom line is health at every size, a paradigm based on behavior, not body-mass index.

"I think it's common sense that people of all sizes, regardless of what they weigh . . . [should] eat their veggies and shake their booty on a regular basis. When you attach health-enhancing behavior to an expectation of weight, you poison the positive relationship to nutrition and fitness."

Maybe that's why, every week, she participates in "Making Waves," what she describes as a swim session for fat women. For ninety minutes, there is lap swimming, then water aerobics and weights. After that, the locker room is one big party, filled with big women chatting and laughing. Wann said it's always a funny moment when a thin woman comes in to suit up. At that instant, slender ladies are not part of the in-crowd.

The role reversal, she said, is rich. Imagine a straight man stumbling upon a Gay Pride parade. A rich heiress stuck in coach on a transcontinental flight. Finally, the person used to living the more comfortable life (in this case, the thin woman) gets a taste of life as an outsider.

One of Wann's friends and colleagues is a plus-sized certified aerobics instructor by the name of Lisa Tealer. In January 1997, Tealer opened the Women of Substance Health Spa in Redwood City, California. Geared toward larger woman but weight-neutral in nature, the spa's guiding philosophy was that it should be a safe space, emotionally and physically. There was no touting of weight-loss products at the front desk. No scale in the locker room! That's like a hospital with no needles! In fact, the locker room was specially designed to be wide and soundly constructed, with individual dressing areas for those who wanted them and signs that read, "Entering body disparagement-free zone" posted throughout. Can you imagine?

Tealer said that sometimes, although not often, locker room dynamics would get "interesting" in that a woman would start talking about dieting or weight-loss surgery . . . things the Women of Substance Health Spa did not promote. So, Tealer said, the club members would have a town meeting of sorts to bring the negative talk out of the locker room and into the open.

As Tealer explained this to me, it sounded like some sort of fictional tale, an anecdote made impossible by social pressures and the First Amendment. But no, it happened, and I think it sounds pretty freaking fabulous.

Unfortunately, because of financial difficulties, the Women of Substance Health Spa closed in 2001. But its legacy lives on: Tealer teaches a class geared toward other plus-sized women called "Great Shape" at a local YMCA. The locker room there, like the one at the club she cofounded, is what she calls a body-image haven.

"It's amazing when you take away those stigmas [of a typical locker room], how freeing it can be," she said. At the Y, there are women of all shapes and sizes, talking and laughing, naked as the day they were born. People have things to talk about besides their thighs and rear ends, such as their jobs, their grandchildren, their vacations. Quite a difference from more traditional gyms, where Tealer sees women "jumping on the scale every five minutes, saying, 'Oh, I had chocolate cake so I can only have salad for dinner.' It's almost a toxic environment, especially if you've been in an environment where that's not an option."

I've never been in a locker room environment where that wasn't an option. And you know what that makes me feel? A few familiar words come to mind.

Disgust
Embarrassment
Sadness
Disappointment
Anxiety
Anger

10

¿Me Veo Gorda en Esta Ropa?
Do I Look Fat in This?

Re-Imagining Body Image:
Exploring Race and Ethnicity

Sometime toward the middle of last summer, I was in the locker room applying a new lotion that had just hit the market. It contained a medium amount of self-tanner as well as those wonderful "conditioning emollients" that would ensure a streakless dark tan. As I massaged the cream into my skin, dreaming of the creamy caramel hue that would develop within four to six hours, I overheard a mother and daughter chatting in a language I thought was Chinese. As I bent down to rub the lotion into my calves, I saw that the two of them were passing a giant-sized bottle of Johnson's Baby Powder between them. (Although the brand name was recognizable, everything else on the product was written in another language, which I would soon come to learn was Thai.) The daughter, who appeared to be my age, was applying the powder in much the way I was applying my lotion, rubbing the silky talc across her shoulders and collarbone and up and down her slender arms.

However, I was using deep circular motions to avoid streaking, but she was extremely light-handed with her application, particularly when it came to her face. Using her first two fingers, she carefully tap, tap, tapped the powder all around as if it were eye cream. It wasn't Kabuki-like, but the point was clear: She was trying to make her naturally olive-toned skin appear lighter. As for me? I was desperate for a cancer-free way to darken my pasty white skin. In fact, just weeks earlier I had stood naked (except for a shower cap) in what was essentially a human car-wash booth, breath held tightly, as jet sprays painted me front and back with ice-cold tanning mist.

The deviation in epidermic desires hit me like a ton of Bobbi Brown Shimmer Bricks: She wanted to be whiter; I longed to be darker. It got me thinking: What other types of cultural, racial, or ethnic divides exist, in the locker room and beyond, when it comes to how we women view our bodies?

Culture Club

If ever a culture chasm exists, it's in the locker room. First of all, at least in my locker room, nearly every member of the housekeeping staff is Latina, and I would guesstimate that less than 5 percent of the actual member pool hails from a minority community (my gym keeps no official record).

Of course, there are members of different races and ethnic backgrounds. There's the black woman with the tiger tattoo on her shoulder blade who, without fail, spends up to twenty minutes meticulously applying this delicious lemon-scented lotion to every inch of her body. Sometimes I arrive and, even if she's not there, I know I must have just missed her because the aroma hangs heavy in the air.

There's a gorgeous older European woman who spends time sauntering from sauna to steam room and back again, luxuriating in the heat. Her deep olive skin drips with sweat, but it's smooth, too, surely belying a childhood spent beneath the hot sun of her childhood country. She converses with her sauna partner, also European—Italian, maybe—in their silky, sexy language, their curly brunette hair piled high atop their heads, but everything waxed smooth down below.

And then there are the white girls. There are many, many white girls. Traditionally, Caucasian women have borne the brunt of society's pressure to be thin, to be tubular except for their breasts, to look like the models in the magazines who are, the majority of the time, white. (Although, thankfully, that is changing, thanks to stereotype breakers such as Tyra Banks and Devon Aoki.) Curves are abhorred, except when artificially gained, as in the case of breast implants.

An example of the powerful pressure of the stereotypical white woman body image: In 1999, the Harvard Eating Disorders Center published a study of Fijian women who, throughout history, have been proud of their fuller figures. For centuries, fat was desired; a drop in weight was a cause for social concern. It meant you were either sick or could not afford to eat enough.

But in 1995, American television shows were introduced to the island. Think *Baywatch* and *Beverly Hills, 90210.* With American TV's arrival came a virtually immediate epidemic of eating problems. Within three years, the number of Fijian teenagers at risk for eating disorders had more than doubled. Of the teenagers surveyed, 74 percent reported that they felt "too big or fat" and 62 percent reported that they had dieted within the past month. Bulimia, a disease never heard of before in Fiji, seemingly appeared out of thin air. This, from a people who, prior to seeing the unattainable images of *Melrose Place* and *Xena, Warrior Princess,* had been proud of their bodies and had striven to avoid weight loss.

My gym recently updated its cardiovascular equipment by installing individual television monitors on much of the equipment. MTV and *Access Hollywood* blare out from the screens, fueling the workouts of everyone there, regardless of race or ethnicity. Whether we are anorexic or obese, apple- or pear-shaped, four foot eight or six foot three, we are caught in an endless cycle of treadmills, Stairmasters, and stationary bikes, running, climbing, and cycling in place for hours to . . . where? To nowhere and everywhere. To the land of thin. Images of Jessica Simpson, J. Lo, and Beyoncé are our equivalent of *Beverly Hills, 90210* in Fiji. After we step off the machines, after the burn from the sit-ups has sufficiently been felt and the stretching is over, we retreat to the locker room. The images linger in our minds like a camera's flash slowly diminishing behind our eyes. But eventually we must open them and we're left staring in the mirror. Or at the women changing next to us. Or at the scale.

Does It Matter If You're Black or White?

When Michael Jackson's pivotal "Black or White" music video premiered in the early 1990s, legions of teenagers nationwide gathered around their televisions to watch the groundbreaking experiment in facial/racial morphing. I know my family was among them. I remember sitting in our kitchen on Ridgewood Lane, watching the perky blonde with the blue eyes and thin nose look to her right and suddenly change into a handsome black man with brown eyes and a broad nose; he, in turn, smiled his way into a Korean woman with swingy black hair and Asian facial features. It was so cool and, at that moment, I knew Michael was right—it don't matter whether you're black or white.

But Jackson was only showing faces. What about the bodies that supported those beautiful but diverse heads? (Of course, these were all actors and probably ridiculously in shape, but let's talk real people.)

For instance, Monica, who is thirty-four and black ("Let's go old school," she said when I asked her how she identifies racially—African American or black), was naturally thin as a child. But when she began attending a more racially diverse high school, she discovered skinniness was an actual goal for some girls. "I guess it's good if you're black—it's nice to be curvy, to have junk in the trunk."

It wasn't until Monica moved out on her own that she started to store some of that junk in *her* trunk. Now, she says she's about 100 pounds overweight, but it hasn't hampered her social life at all. Men still hit her up for her phone number—black men, that is. Maybe if she had her sights set on a white man, she hypothesized, "it would be a problem."

Pardon the pun, but it would be a *really big* problem.

Consider Dove's ingenious summer 2005 media campaign, which featured real women of all sizes and races posing and laughing in their white cotton underwear (versus stick-thin models staring seductively and, I would imagine, hungrily, into the camera's lens). The ads sparked a firestorm of newspaper editorials and cocktail party conversation in which women fought bleached tooth and manicured nail to defend the ads; men (and I'll just speak for the men I overheard, who were white) made comments ranging from "Oh, are you talking about that the new ad for big chicks?" to "Ugh, I don't wanna see that!" (Guess what, little guy: We don't want to see your man boobs and spare tire, but you don't hear us complaining in public forums, do you? That's right. Now go wax your back.)

Monica works out about four times a week and would like to try to lose some weight but thinks a regimented diet would stress her out, which isn't her style. So she's taking it as it comes. But she was unpleasantly surprised when, after a recent aerobics class, she encountered her very own Cheryl Peck moment. After class, which she completed successfully, thankyouverymuch, a fellow gym-goer approached Monica to compliment her on a job well done. The underlying message came through loud and clear: You did well . . . for an overweight person.

I would like to take a moment to point out that it wasn't until about halfway into our conversation that Monica even mentioned the fact that she is 100 pounds overweight. As a woman who for years has planned her lunches around what she's eating for dinner, this blows my mind.

But that isn't to say that issues of body image aren't on Monica's radar or that African American girls don't struggle with body-image issues. Just a couple of months after we first spoke, she sent me a link to a *New York Times* story titled "Blacks Join the Eating-Disorder Mainstream." The piece started with an interview with a young African American woman who recounted her battle with bulimia, which began in high school when she was one of nine black students in a school of three thousand. Her perception of beauty, she explained, was based on what she saw: white peers and white celebrities.

Janet, twenty-five, a black medical student, describes herself as falling somewhere between thin and heavy on the weight spectrum. But when conducting a research project on Body Mass Index, she found her BMI teetering on overweight. "If I were to ask my mom if I was overweight, she'd say I was fine," said Janet, who works out fairly regularly. And although she knows the United States, as a whole, is obese, she acknowledged that many women in the black community are not only praised for their curves—hence the incongruity between how Janet views her body shape and where the BMI places her—but "it's more accepted to be overweight than to be underweight, whereas in the white community, you may be pushed to be thin."

Janet's medical background is evident in her comments about being in the locker room: She said she finds it interesting to see how differently all women are put together in terms of body type. She doesn't compare herself to others, regardless of their race or ethnicity; rather, she said she finds it comforting to see real women of all color who "have cellulite, who have droopy things, who have pudgy stomachs." Physical quirks that don't discriminate.

Twenty-two-year-old LaMecia, also black, didn't react nearly as well to her BMI measurement, however; in fact, it almost drove her to an eating disorder. Standing nearly five foot nine, sporting large thigh and calf muscles but without a well-defined waist, LaMecia was always active in sports, including cheerleading, track, and swimming, but she was also one of the heaviest of her friends. Her family was always supportive of her physical fitness and the fit, strong figure that came with it. But when her doctor measured her BMI as a teenager and deemed her overweight, LaMecia launched herself into a dietary program that included school lunches composed solely of sodas and small bags of chips. Even though the food was unhealthy, the decreased calories combined with all of her activity helped her drop from 165 pounds to 135.

But she said she now thinks her old photos show her looking "emaciated." Although that height and weight might be desirable in certain ethnic groups, it didn't fly in a culture where it's okay to have meat on your bones. So in her senior year, she quit a few sports and was able to gain back about 20 pounds. The result: a better, "thicker" LaMecia.

The "thicker" LaMecia (whose weight actually still falls within the parameters of "normal") now finds herself enjoying life much more, and she even takes the occasional opportunity to conduct a bit of informal diversity education with friends. For example, when she attended an NFL game last fall with a group of multiracial friends, a black girl with a touchdown-inspiring booty walked by, leaving one white male friend with his jaw to the turf.

"We had to explain to them it was okay," she said with a chuckle. "Some of [them] were like, 'Oh, really?'"

LaMecia thinks the whole "big butt" phenomenon and its more general acceptance in the black community can be attributed in part to its appeal to the opposite sex. Being bigger, she said, shows men not only that you are healthy but also "that you can eat and can probably cook." Thinking back to the days when her tall, muscular frame bore only 135 pounds, she certainly didn't appear healthy, let alone ready to prepare a home-cooked meal. Today, she stands firm in her decision that she "never wants to be that thin again, never wants to go back there again."

We Are Barbie Girls

If LaMecia looked "emaciated" at five foot nine and 135 pounds, why is it that no one uttered a peep when I starved myself down to that weight—and I'm nearly two inches taller? Maybe because in the Caucasian community, "emaciation" has been accepted, even been encouraged? Never mind the fact that dogs of certain breeds weigh more than 135 pounds. When I was sick, girls in my dorm (99.9 percent of them white) asked me for weight-loss tips; guys asked me out on dates. It wasn't until I reached that tipping point of 130 pounds that people started to become concerned. And I became a cliché. The white, first-born, overachieving, middle-to-upper-class anorexic. How boringly formulaic.

My friend Amanda (of Crabwalk fame) believes her prior eating disorder and current struggle to accept her beautiful— but no longer stick-thin—body originated long ago. When she was growing up in the 1980s, she remembered, "the media, the fashion magazines, they all focused on white women, who were glamorous and thin." She added, "I started forming my sense of what was acceptable in terms of weight by that." Now, with more attention paid to women of color in the media, Amanda feels the general message drifting toward accepting one's body; but with white women, she said, "it's never about acceptance."

As the prototypical blonde-haired, blue-eyed, Swedish bikini-team girl (and she really is Swedish), Amanda admitted she feels pressure, a sense of responsibility to carry off the "All-American Beauty" image that comes from society, from the opposite sex, even from her family. She used to exercise compulsively; now, as the co-owner of a beauty shop (where the walls are, ironically, painted with witticisms such as "A well-groomed girl is a well-adjusted girl"), she simply doesn't have enough time to devote hours to the gym. So she walks a few miles to work and back, donning $200+ "anti-cellulite sneakers"—so long as her outfit allows it, fashionably speaking.

At her furniture-store side job, one Latina coworker takes great joy in occasionally telling Amanda that she has a big ass "for a white girl." But she doesn't mean it as an insult. In her community, a curvy rear is a good thing. But the coworker has no idea that Amanda suffers body-image woes, no clue that her remarks sting Amanda inside. And can you imagine how that would go over if it was one white woman saying it to another? Deadpanned Amanda, "I would never tell one of my white girlfriends she had a big ass. I'd be slapped."

Who You Callin' Jaadi?

Lina's problem was the opposite of Monica's: She was overweight as a child, but thinned out as an adult. Unfortunately, she failed to escape the traditional Indian nickname "Jaadi," a teasing but lovable term that means "fatso." When she was six, the nickname was used mostly by her aunts and uncles, but it stuck with her through junior high.

In high school, Lina, now thirty-one, began to shed her baby fat through track and pom-poms—so much so that by her senior year her sister became concerned that she was losing too much weight; she thought that perhaps "Jaadi" was heading for an eating disorder because at dinner, if she had one carb, such as rice, she would skip the roti (a type of Indian flat bread).

But by college, everything leveled out. Lina settled into a healthy weight and chose a major: nutrition. Although she had never suffered an eating disorder, she recalled poll results that found that 80 percent of students in one of her nutrition classes had a history of eating disorders. (Jesus, will somebody develop some sort of screening process for this major already?)

Now, at five foot two, Lina fluctuates between a size 0 and a size 4. She works out a lot but can clean a plate with the best of them. She's one of those women about whom people gripe, "I can't believe how much you can get away with eating."

There are two other Indian women Lina knows of who work out at her gym. She's fairly modest while changing, which she believes comes partly from her Indian culture. As an example, kissing in movies has just been introduced in her family's home country. But to provide an interesting contrast, she pointed out that although a traditional Indian sari consists of nine feet of fabric, the midriff is always showing, no matter what shape, size, or age the wearer, and the cloth comes to just under the breasts. In fact, large breasts and a voluptuous stomach customarily have been praised on an Indian woman as symbols of fertility—no firming push-ups or crunches necessary.

However, with the advent of Bollywood (very risqué, ornate Indian films), the bar has been raised for Indian actresses in America to shed pounds, and every day women are following suit. Thin is in for younger Indian American women, Lina said. Welcome to the club.

You Can Do Side-Bends or Sit-Ups, but Please Don't Lose That Butt

No clearer was the wild cultural divergence in body-type preference made than during a recent trip to South Beach, perhaps the most body-obsessed U.S. city ever (Los Angeles is just too fake to count). Walking down the main strip, my husband's friend made the rather astute observation that the mannequins' butts and thighs were all much, much larger than those seen in our hometown of Chicago. In his skillful, rum-laced words, "Me likey." But wait . . . I thought we women were supposed to be working our asses off—literally—in the gym? Now I come to find out that all I have to do is migrate south, where rump reigns and I can toss my running shoes? Can't a girl catch a frigging break? Why is it that the Dove girls with ample curves, who are soft all over, get shunned by men, but a few well-placed semicircles stuck on an otherwise lithe frame leave men drowning in a puddle of their own drool?

As it turns out, the mannequins we were gawking at were likely part of the 2003 "Sex" line, created by one of the nation's foremost mannequin manufacturers, Goldsmith. The line was designed in response to the nation's shifting gaze toward a fuller rear, inspired by Jennifer Lopez's much-lauded backside. One of the foremost role models for Latinas today, J. Lo rocks a curvy rear and hips, but she must exercise pretty damned hard for those washboard abs and sleek dancer's legs.

My friend Veronica, thirty, who told me that when she joined her health club she was "the only nonwhite person in the locker room besides the cleaning lady," thinks J. Lo's butt is overrated. Veronica is Mexican, but she said curves are still essential. As long as your butt looks good in jeans and you're set in the chest department, you're good to go, she told me. "If I didn't have that, my mom would probably tell me I looked sick, like I needed meat on my bones."

Veronica thinks women like my (white) friends are crazy for exercising most days and then feeling guilty about missing a workout. People in her culture tend not to get obsessed, she said. "It's like, 'I'll get to it when I can.'" (This type of attitude is refreshing from a body-image viewpoint, but it can also be dangerous. According to the National Diabetes Information Clearinghouse, obesity-induced diabetes is rampant in the Hispanic community.)

When she can make it, however, the locker room is much different for Veronica than for, say, a gringa like me. She recalled hitting the showers with a white former coworker who preferred to walk around naked, no towel necessary. For someone raised in a culture where modesty rules, watching a colleague stroll about in her birthday suit was too much for Veronica to bear.

"She was talking to me, moving her arms, and her boobs were flapping everywhere," Vero recalled. "She was like, 'What's wrong? We're both women, we have the same things.' I made up some excuse about my stomach being so damaged by the stretch marks from my pregnancy—which it is. When I showed her, her reaction was ridiculous, freaking out." Gee, that must've done a lot to make Veronica want to blow-dry her hair *desnuda.*

Today, Veronica continues to change in the shower, drying off and putting on fresh undies and bra before emerging wrapped in a towel. "It's a cultural thing," she explained. "A lot of my friends do it, too."

But as Alma, also Latina, pointed out, Hispanic women—just like any other ethnic group—are highly individualized when it comes to body-image issues. For instance, this thirty-four-year-old with "more of a chest than an ass" works out about four times a week and changes out in the open, even though her locker room offers individualized changing rooms. Much like Veronica's flapping-breast coworker, Alma "figures everyone there has the same stuff," although she does sometimes think she's being watched by some of the heavier women, that someone's looking a little longer than they should.

Alma talked about an inner drive she feels to look a certain way and was the first woman I'd spoken with to bring up the possibility that not all Latinas or black women feel comfortable being curvier or heavier. The stereotype is pervasive, she acknowledged, and, to a large extent, accepted, but that doesn't mean she looks at it that way.

A False Sense of Safety

Although this wasn't the case with the majority of the women profiled here, Becky Thompson, PhD, author of *A Hunger So Wide and So Deep,* spoke with eighteen women of different racial and ethnic backgrounds and found the belief that blacks and Latinas are somehow protected from eating disorders to be a dangerous fallacy. Dr. Thompson found that although the media does play a role, she heard tales of trauma and loss from women of color that extended way beyond the influence of magazine advertisements or movie-star experiences. Sexual abuse, racism, fear of coming out of the closet, losing a parent, and not fitting in as an immigrant were all factors cited as playing a role in eating disorders, whether that meant denying food as a way to gain control or using food as comfort.

"This whole idea that black and Latina women don't develop eating problems frightens me because it suggests we live in other universes," said Dr. Thompson, who is white. Just because these ladies are watching white women "getting on the scale four times a day" doesn't mean they're not doing it themselves, she said—"they may just be doing it in other places. It's just more underground."

She also pointed out that weight is only one type of "Geiger counter" used to measure women's body image. For white women, it may be the most prominent one; but for black and Latina women, there's skin color, hair texture, and bone structure. LaMecia, the young lady from above who dieted after a disappointing BMI, mentioned that her lighter skin tone has been an issue all her life. She's been referred to as "yellow," the meaning of which at times has been complimentary and at other times demeaning. Lina also said that in the Indian culture, skin tone carries an impact. For her community, "the fairer you are, the better."

Dealing with Different Ends of the Rainbow

I met Shannon during college, when she was the director of advertising for our university's paper. About five years ago,

Shannon was hostessing at one of the hippest restaurants in New York City when Tommy Mattola and Marc Anthony came in to dine. Halfway through their meal, they invited Shannon over, complimented her on her exotic beauty, and asked her to appear in one of Anthony's upcoming videos. And wouldn't you know it but two weeks later that lucky lady was flying in first class next to Marc himself on their way to Rio de Janeiro, where she was paid some ridiculous amount of money to get pampered, massaged, and eventually to dress up—not as a video ho but as a *hotel worker*, fully clothed, for six hours in front of the camera.

Not that I blame the power boys for being attracted to her. At five foot eleven and a sleek size 8, Shannon has creamy latte-colored skin and delicate features, the beautiful creation of a West Indian mother who hails from Guyana, a tropical country located on the northeast coast of South America, and a Scottish father. But growing up as a biracial child wasn't all peaches and cream. In fact, it was downright confusing at times for Shannon.

On her mother's side, the women were voluptuous and curvy, and food was always the focal point of family gatherings. Body size was never the main topic of discussion.

But when it came to get-togethers with her father's side of the family, including her dad's six sisters, who were petite in stature and constantly comparing themselves to one another, it was a different story. "It was always about the body," Shannon said. "When they served food, it was always very small portions and they'd be eating like birds." Whereas on her mom's side, the portions were humongous, often two to three servings each. Naturally tall and slender, Shannon found herself caught in a family no-(wo)man's land: Given a hard time that she should eat more and more by her mom's side, praised for her slim build by her aunts on her dad's side.

Ultimately, she chose to identify with her mother's outlook on body image because "it was just less stressful," she said. "My mom's side focused on being happy and spending time together." As a result, she believes, she has a positive sense of self today and feels good in her skin. She'd rather be strong and healthy than slim and unfit.

Shannon works out with a trainer at a gym popular with models—*Elite* sends their girls there, she said. So being in the locker room was initially a bit jolting because of their (lack of) size. "I felt like they would assume other women wanted to be their size," Shannon said, "and I wanted to wear a T-shirt that said, 'I Don't Want to Look Like You, Because You Look Hungry!'"

J. Mori, thirty-five, of African and Asian descent, is another biracial woman who has grappled with her body image as a result of her dual-ethnic identity. Her mom is Japanese, stands four foot eight, and, while raising J. Mori, weighed an amount I could probably bench-press; her father is black, five foot eight, and just 120 pounds. Next to me, they would seem downright Lilliputian. J. Mori said she was fortunate in that she was raised in a household where being naked was not something to be ashamed of. If she accidentally saw one of her parents in the buff, it was nothing to write into a teen magazine's "Most embarrassing moments" page about.

But once puberty, lovely puberty hit, J. Mori was confronted with a number of body-image issues. First of all, she said, her mom is "pretty much hairless," which was an issue because J. Mori did have a lot of body hair, forcing her to look to the women on her father's side for advice. Another thing: J. Mori had always assumed that because her mom had DD boobs, she would be stacked, too. But once she started changing in the middle school locker room, it became painfully apparent to this active tomboy that although the other girls' breasts were starting to develop, hers were still in hibernation mode.

As a teenager, she grew up in a multicultural community where multiple body types were accepted, so she wasn't self-conscious about changing clothes at school. But she definitely saw that her black and Hispanic girlfriends were more voluptuous and curvy. "They had bigger butts, bigger thighs, hips," she said, "and my white friends were thinner and taller. I just jumped to the conclusion that everyone was built differently. We would joke around in the locker room. This white girl, Tori, we would tease her that she was part black because her butt was kind of big. It was that kind of stereotypical teasing. There were lots of people like me—interracial, as well as multicultural. So I took it for granted . . . I never had any issues of, 'Why don't I look like this or that?'"

It wasn't until J. Mori began college that she started "filling out." Whether it was the Freshman 15 or going on birth control, she does not know what prompted the weight gain, but she does know that it was *all good*. She received ample attention from black men and began to get interested in makeup and tight jeans; she would perk up when black men made positive comments about her being "thick"—and this is coming from a woman who had been very tomboyish and had cared little about trivial matters such as clothes, dating, and cosmetics. The increased attention, she said, made her feel very sexy.

Today, she belongs to a gym in which she is one of two women of color; the rest of the females are white, and most of them, she said, are "definitely skinnier." Although she recognizes that she likely falls on the heavier end of the spectrum, she remains confident. She and her friends talk about working out for the sake of being healthy and fit, not to lose weight.

Despite her confidence, J. Mori does notice that the women in her gym tend to dress a bit more scantily, in a sports bra and shorts, for example, or even, yes, a leotard thong over bike shorts. J. Mori sticks to T-shirts and sweats, as does the other black woman at her club. She finds the contradiction intriguing.

"It's interesting that for women who are supposed to be a little more comfortable with their bodies, we don't try to show our bodies off. It's like we're personally comfortable but not publicly comfortable." She wondered whether perhaps she still feels that larger societal force saying she is bigger than she should be.

But then that societal force seemingly disappeared when she told me about her recreational volleyball league, noticeably absent of minorities. While playing, J. Mori dons a T-shirt, but the other girls wear bikinis. "Do they have good bodies?" I asked J. Mori, to which she responded, "Well, that depends on what you consider a good body. I guess you could say yes, in that they're thin and tiny but no, it's not the body type I would find most attractive."

Running the Joint

Because most members of the locker room staff at my gym are Latina, I was itching to speak with them about what it was like to be on "the other side." After all, most of them are quite voluptuous, and they are confronted, day in and day out, with a rather obsessive clientele. Not just obsessive, but naked and obsessive. Always a winning combination.

Every one of the staff members is always pleasant and courteous to me, even though a breast is often popping out of my towel as I pass by, or my hair is so soaked with sweat that even though I've untied it, it's still quite content to remain in ponytail position. Bottom line, I'm not a pretty sight. Still, they smile and nod as I grab an extra towel and head for the showers (many of them do not speak English). But I always wondered, "Do they think I'm this crazy white girl who works out all the time and is obsessed with her body?" After all, the closest most of them come to the gigantic Toledo scale is the phone situated immediately next to it, where many of them make and receive calls while on break.

Maria, sixty, has been working at the gym for twenty-six years. The den mother of the locker room, she looks far younger than her age and always has an easy grin on her face. With light, barely wrinkled skin and a caring demeanor, Maria has handed me Band-Aids for my shaving cuts and always says hello and goodbye to me. But it wasn't until we sat down at the hairstyling station that I learned she was bilingual.

When I asked her about some of the body-image-related things she's seen in our locker room over the decades, Maria recalled a woman who used to work out at our gym. She was white, a woman who had "a little more meat" on her, motioning to her waist—but she did so in a nonjudgmental, almost complimentary way. But after five or six years, the woman began losing weight. "You could see her ribs, her spinal column. Sometimes she'd stay in the whirlpool for two hours—she'd fall asleep and I'd have to wake her up," Maria said, her eyes widening. She didn't know what happened to that lady. Who knows what happens to so many of them?

Mireya, fifty-two, joined us, and Maria translated for her: "How do Hispanic women and white women seem to differ in their body images?" I asked. They conversed in Spanish for a bit and Maria turned to me and reported, "She says, '[White women] want to be so skinny and lose so much weight. It's like,'" and she struggled with the word that rolls so easily off America's collective tongue, "'anorexia.'"

Maria grew up in Puerto Rico, where her mother taught her always to cover herself. Even shorts were off-limits. So when she began working at my gym, it was quite a shock to see women walking around topless, or even totally nude.

"I thought, 'Why don't they cover up?' There are children in here," Maria recalled. Even now, she's not completely comfortable with it—she tries to avert her eyes. I felt a pang of guilt, because I've probably said hello to Maria about a thousand times while topless. Won't be doing that anymore.

I asked another locker room staffer whether they chat about us, fully expecting her to answer in the affirmative. How could they not? And in fact, she said they do, but her reasoning surprised me. "Yes, sometimes," she said. "Like when they're big and they keep coming and coming but they don't lose." (She preferred to remain nameless.) Also, some of the older staff members think the thongs so many of us wear look uncomfortable. I don't think that's a cultural thing, though, but rather a generational issue.

Carmen, twenty-six, moved here five years ago from El Salvador. Her interview had to be translated by Esmerelda, also twenty-six, who has lived here all her life. I asked Carmen whether she thinks the mostly white clientele seems to focus excessively on weight. She responded shyly, "You guys look nice. Thin. Maybe obsessed with being thin." I asked about our fixation with the scale, to which Carmen replied, "If it makes you feel better about yourselves every time you come in to see if you lost a pound or more, it's okay." For some reason, I wasn't sure I believed her, so I probed a bit deeper and asked Esmerelda to inquire once more. That's when Carmen admitted, "No, it's kind of strange. Kind of like an obsession. To me, it seems like you want to lose lots more weight when you're already at a small size."

The answers changed a bit when Esmerelda, fluent in English, was the one doing the talking; her answers came across as completely uninhibited. Having been raised in the United States and now working in a mostly white locker room, she said she is hit hard by the pressure to lose weight. But for her, the pressure comes from within. (Although, she said, eating disorders are an issue in Mexico, where her family comes from—especially in the capital. Women there use bulimia as a way to maintain their curves—but not get *too* curvy—while still eating, she explained.) Esmerelda has just given birth to her third baby and hasn't been able to shed all the weight, which frustrates her. She finds herself getting on the scale often to track her progress.

"It bothers me that I can't lose weight like . . ." she said, and then motioned up and down to me. I realized she meant this as a compliment to me, but she was actually insulting herself. I mean, there was a fundamental difference—she had just given birth to her *third baby;* the last thing I delivered was my Visa payment to the mailbox. And, unlike her, I've had an eating disorder. I've been one of those ladies in the Mexican capital making themselves throw up. She hasn't. So for me, striving to stay thin has been more of a necessary evil in my life, fed by societal pressures, whereas in her community, being curvy is generally more acceptable—hell, more desired—although eating disorders are on the rise. Meanwhile, she said, she and the other staff members watch as I and the other "younger white females look in the mirror and say, 'Ooh, my butt needs to look tighter.'" Esmerelda said this in a sort of mocking falsetto, implying that most of our butts do not.

As for the nudity issue, it appears that, across the board, all Latina staff members I spoke with were brought up with a heavy degree of modesty. Explained Esmerelda, "In my house, my mom never talked about my breasts growing in or that I'm going to start to develop. But when I came here [to the heath club] women seemed so liberal, so free. They just walk around showing everything. Sometimes it's pretty weird because they just bend over and show everything and for me, it's like, 'Oh my God!'"

So now I'll know, the next time I hear someone exclaim *"Ay dios mio!"* I'm probably giving someone a money shot. That's the kind of lesson in multiculturalism you just can't get in school.

11

The Next Generation

*Body Image, Locker Room Mentality,
and Today's Young Girls*

In the fifth grade, Meghan was the leader of her very popular clique. The Queen Bee, if you will. If she stopped to take a drink from the water fountain, all the girls stopped. If she bent over to tie her shoelace, the troops waited patiently for the perfect bow to be knotted.

The fifth grade was a good time to be Meghan.

But things changed during the summer between fifth and sixth grade. Meghan's "right hand girl" began, shall we say, maturing; hanging out with boys and doing things that, apparently—sadly—many soon-to-be sixth-grade girls do with boys these days. Such as drinking. Drugs. Oral sex. But Meghan didn't want to do those things. So the girl who used to be her best friend got together with some of the other young ladies and drew up a list of ultimatums, things Meghan would have to do if she wanted to stay cool. Such as drinking. Drugs. Oral sex. Meghan stood her ground, and the soldierettes who used to walk on eggshells around her promptly proceeded to stomp on her reputation, reducing her self-esteem to precisely that: eggshells.

The sixth grade was not a good time to be Meghan. With virtually the entire grade turned against her, school was hell. Gym class was especially tortuous. Besides the typical agony that comes with changing in a junior high locker room, she had to deal with her peers' unrelenting taunting and teasing. Someone had scrawled "PIG" across Meghan's desk—even though she was by no means overweight—which sent her scurrying for the bathroom stalls to change. But even those metal walls provided no safe haven. Day in and day out, as Meghan hurriedly attempted to change into her gym uniform, locked in the bathroom stall like some sort of caged animal, those sixth-grade bullies would kick the doors open, laughing, just to catch her mid-change.

Not surprisingly, Meghan developed an eating disorder as a way to cope with her extremely disordered school life. "I remember going home one day and looking in the mirror and seeing a totally different Meghan," she told me. "I wanted to just break my mirror. I was like, 'I'm just not going to eat any more.'"

Luckily, the harassment abated over the next year or so as the girls lost interest in their target. As their persecution waned, Meghan's eating habits normalized. She also found theater, which provided her with an outlet for her emotions. Today, at sixteen, she is a gorgeous sophomore, with doe eyes and a heart-shaped face framed by long brunette locks. Tall and fawn-like, she has the legs of a mini-Rockette, which she displays in a skirt just a few inches shorter than my laptop. She is beautiful and I feel badly for the boys because she is gonna be a heartbreaker (if she isn't already).

I asked Meghan what her favorite part of her body is. "My legs," she replied with a smile. No surprise there. Her least favorite? "My tummy."

Pause.

"Because it's there."

She still changes in the bathroom stall during gym class.

Meghan was concerned about coming off as a weight-obsessed young woman in this book. "I'm very proud of myself, of my personality," she said. "I have great friends. I'm one of those people who could definitely get on the table with a boa and dance." But, she added, there is one caveat. "If people call me fat, I can't take it."

High School Homecoming

In 2000, I began volunteering my services as a public speaker, visiting high schools, colleges, and medical schools to talk about what life is like with anorexia. My first stop on the tour, for whatever bizarre, subconscious reasons, was my suburban high school. Why, I have no idea. I don't harbor particularly fond memories of high school. Although I was an A student and had a close group of friends, I spent the better part of it dodging nasty names by the "popular" girls (most of whom ended up knocked up and never finished college, I might happily add) because I was popular with the boys, whom I dated extensively but never let get past second base.

And I was a flag girl during my sophomore year, okay?

But no need to dwell.

So I had this wealth of knowledge about eating disorders that I wanted to share with the younger generation. I contacted my former high school health teacher and, before I knew it, I was back at my old alma mater—in my high school locker room, in fact. I crouched down to apply my lipstick in a mirror anchored way too low for my tall self as I prepared to deliver a speech eight straight times to eight straight periods of high school sophomores. I had already peeked into the classroom to survey my audience, and I was horrified at how . . . well, how mature the girls looked. How these poor, acne-riddled boys suppressed their omnipresent erections was far beyond me. Did we wear halter tops to class in 1992? Flippy little skirts with ruffles? Heels?! I'm all for individuality, but I asked the football coach who was with me whether there was some sort of dress code. These weren't girls, they were miniature women; and the boys, with their braces and unwashed hair, were so clearly still boys. Coach told me that during the section on first aid, they would make the girls tie varsity football jackets around their waists as they pump, pump, pumped life back into the mannequin-cadavers, lest their skirts flip up and the boys' penises spring skyward, knocking them unconscious. Clearly, these girls were in a hurry to grow up—or were at least dressing in an attempt to keep pace with their fast-maturing bodies.

I would speak, no holds barred, about my experience with an eating disorder. I told them about my goody-goody days of high school, right in these very classrooms. About my earliest weeks of college, when, at my first frat party, I saw a gaggle of girls from the East Coast, all stick-thin and glossy black hair and no hips and how I vowed that the next day I would start running more, just to lose a few pounds and tone up. And how that turned into midnight hour-long runs across campus and lunches of lettuce and salsa and guilt-induced near-purges because I ate the tip—the tip!—off of a Hershey's Kiss.

I told them how I lost my breasts and my period and about the first time my boyfriend realized I didn't wear a bra. How my cheeks and under eyes sunk inward and my watch would slide perilously close to my elbow. How I would log endless hours studying in the library, taking breaks with my expensive graphing calculator to add up the number of calories I had taken in that day, praying that, when I hit the "total" button, it wasn't more than eight hundred.

As I spoke, some girls filed their nails or passed notes back and forth. Others stared at me with wide eyes, soaking in each word like a sponge. The boys? Perhaps it was awkward for them, hearing me talk about periods and boobs and throwing up (I dabbled in that for a short time, too), but I stressed to them that I could easily be their sister or girlfriend. After all, I told them (perhaps to the chagrin of the teachers), when my college boyfriend first reached under my shirt to find I went bra-less, he had no clue I had an eating disorder; he simply thought I was cool.

Inevitably, after each fifty-minute period, when that bell rang, I would literally be swarmed by masses of girls, some clinging to me as if their lives depended on it, others standing in the background, clutching their books to their chests as they silently waited their turn. Tears streamed down cheeks as students told me stories of boyfriends who called them cows, of fellow female students who made fun of their bodies in the locker room, of magazine advertisements that, try as they might, they feared they would never be able to live up to.

Later, I would gut-wrenchingly learn from Ilana, eighteen, and young ladies like her, that I had simultaneously managed to act as a catalyst for some girls' already budding eating disorders. Ilana, who was obese as a child, told me she had actually learned how to be anorexic and bulimic from recovering women like myself who came and spoke to their health classes. I suppose that shouldn't surprise me, considering I sometimes received e-mails from students, such as one foreign-exchange student from Japan who, not having mastered the English language yet, thanked me for my talk and then explained she just wanted to lose about 10 more pounds but couldn't make herself "Bolivia." I'm not recounting this to make fun of her; just to show how far-reaching the epidemic is.

I remember one girl in particular who approached me after my talk, seeking comfort: Short and cute in her denim overalls, her clear blue eyes swollen and red. Strands of her long blonde hair stuck to her damp cheeks and lips as she cried. Her boyfriend was calling her names, she confided in me.

"Names like what?" I asked her, pulling the wet hair out of her glassy, ocean-colored eyes and tucking it behind her ears.

"F-f-fat," she managed to escape between wet sobs.

When you're fifteen and vulnerable and living in today's society, can anything be worse?

Setting an Example

When it comes to today's teenage girl, the locker room experience is usually limited to two places. First, the school locker room, where she is either being teased, doing the tormenting, or simply minding her own business and getting in and out of her gym uniform as fast as possible (although some, like Fiona, a fifteen-year-old water polo player, are blessedly nonchalant: "Everyone has seen everything on each other and no one cares anymore," she explained). But my research, both anecdotal and personal, tells me that Fiona is in the minority. Girls *do* care. Every grown woman I know has at least a handful of vivid middle school or high school memories of the locker room burned into her mind, from desperately trying to hide her training bra from the more developed girls, to showering in an open room with her swimsuit still on, to attempting to mask the crackle of her pad wrapper as she fumbles with it during her first period.

Second, more and more girls are joining health clubs. According to the International Health, Racquet & Sportsclub Association, in 2003 (the latest year for which figures are available), 4.5 million health club memberships belonged to children under the age of eighteen—a 223 percent increase from 1987. That's a lot of young ladies hitting the gym . . . and a lot of teenagers making their entrée into the big-girl world of locker rooms.

In *Dedication to Hunger: The Anorexic Aesthetic in Modern Culture,* competitive athlete turned academic Leslie Heywood opens the book by recounting an afternoon in her locker room. Two young girls nearby are discussing the length of their workout when one of them suddenly turns to Heywood and pleads, "Tell me the truth. The real truth. I want to know. Look at my body. I'm fat. I need to lose weight, don't I?"

The author, having previously battled her own body-image demons, struggles between reassuring the girl of her beauty, while trying to silence her old inner voices aching to agree: "Yes . . . you're not quite linear, not quite a straight line." Heywood's positive reassurance, of course, won out in then end, but she feared it rang hollow.

Who knows what became of that thirteen-year-old, so terrified of her own changing body that she begged a stranger for reassurance, for womanly comfort and solidarity of the most bizarre kind? Considering that I, like her, have demanded that same confirmation—"I'm fat, aren't I?"—from family, friends, and strangers alike at different points in my lifetime, I suspect that she went on to develop some sort of dangerous eating pattern. I hope she proved us wrong.

Negotiating my locker room when there are younger girls around, be they teenagers or pre-teenagers, has always been a tricky experience for me. Part of me wants to shield them from the grown-up aspects of my usual locker room customs, perhaps in an effort to help them stay young and free from body-image issues for just a few more weeks/months/years. Maybe I should cover up my body in the steam room or while en route to the shower so that they don't feel uncomfortable seeing my . . . whatever. Perhaps I should shimmy my thong on underneath my towel so they don't get the idea that they, too, should be wearing G-strings instead of bikini briefs. Or, as the case was on a recent weekend evening, should I really have pulled on that sexy top over a push-up bra and then, using my hands, individually lifted each breast just a bit higher for a more cleavage-y look with youngsters watching me like a hawk? I mean, what kind of harlot am I?

On the other hand, I just want to behave normally, changing at a regular pace with no variations to my normal routine. That may mean showing off a runway bikini line, or hiking my boobs up in my push-up bra, left then right, to make my Bs look a little more C-ish. I'm a grown woman and these are things that grown women do.

But after speaking with a number of teenaged girls, I now realize that much of my worrying has been for naught. As it turns out, many of them are not paying attention to *me*. Rather, they're too busy comparing themselves to each other, to the images they see on television, and to the It Girls their male counterparts drool over. Much to their parents' dismay, I'm sure, my thong is nothing new to them; many of them have collections that would rival mine. Rana, a sixteen-year-old Jewel look-alike whom I approached in my locker room after overhearing her talking with a friend about Clinique mascara, used to change for gym in a bathroom stall because she wears skimpy under-things and didn't want the other girls to see. She doesn't use the stalls to change anymore, but she said other girls literally line up to use them for undressing purposes, even if means making them late for class.

Also, like women of my age, they get bikini waxes. Often, this is not of their own volition: Guys tell them they won't be into fooling around with them unless they're, and I quote, "cleaned up down there." Sometimes, these girls shave *everything,* especially before major occasions. One sixteen-year-old had this request made of her, or shall I say this mandate imposed on her, by her date prior to a prom. She complied, assuring me it wasn't a big deal. (When she told me this, it was all I could do to stop myself from breaking out into sobs. All I can say is, first, I hope her prom date is one day asked by a girlfriend to have his back waxed—and feels every single hair follicle being ripped out individually and, second, I pray the sixteen-year-old had some TendSkin and a good, soft Loofah at home.)

These girls pierce their navels and decorate them with dangling jeweled cherries or pink hearts. They have tattoos of butterflies and fairies sprinkled across the concave of their lower backs. They work out in short shorts with the word "JUICY," "FLIRT," or "PINK" scrawled across their tushes, and they leave grown men salivating in their fruity perfumed wakes. They jump on the scale day in and day out, but much of the time, they follow up a workout with pizza and Cokes. Their teenaged metabolisms and after-school activities just zap the calories away.

My First Gym

Ahh, yes. I remember those days. As a sophomore in high school, I joined my grandfather's gym, which was a big deal at the time because it was where Michael Jordan and the Chicago Bulls practiced. It was an extremely posh gym with a mostly older clientele, and as one of a handful of the younger members, I thought I was a Venti cup of hot shit at that health club. High-impact aerobics followed by three miles on the treadmill and half an hour of weights, all in my midriff-baring tank and bike shorts; I may not have known what a bikini wax was yet, but I knew what a bikini was, and I thought (actually, prayed) that I looked good in one.

But you know, it's funny because upon reflection, I don't have a multitude of striking reflections regarding that particular locker room. Sure, I remember seeing lots of senior-aged women naked, and I remember hopping on the scale every time I was there, but I have many more memories relating to the men among whom I worked out and how they shaped my self-image. In fact, I believe it was *outside* of that ladies' locker room where some of the first seeds of my eating disorder were planted.

I remember one guy, a married man in his early forties, who was always hitting on me in very explicit, inappropriate ways. I'd be sweating it out on the stair machine and he'd come up to make small talk; then suddenly he would switch gears, launching into a detailed breakdown of my body. I remember it, clear as day, wearing a cantaloupe-colored sports bra and heather-gray sweatpants cut off into shorts:

"Your breasts are perfect," he'd say. "Your stomach is so tight, your ass is spectacular."

I was sixteen.

As this man dissected me like a cadaver on a slab of steel, I could do nothing but smile bashfully, assuming this was okay—that I should be proud, even—when really what I should have been doing was calling his wife. These were not compliments; they were uninvited, pedophilic harassments. And yet, they played a pivotal role in molding my self-image: I was just a sum of parts to be ogled by men.

Rana said the same type of thing is still going on today, but the culprits aren't just forty-year-old men; they're high school boys. "They'll make lists of the most attractive girls [in school]," she said. "They might be ranked, like 'Nice butt, but that girl's boobs and face are better.'" Charming.

Katie

Katie was one of the first girls I spoke with regarding body image and the locker room. At seventeen, this suburban high school junior fills her afternoons and weekends with Varsity Poms and Dance Club activities, including ballet, hip hop, tap, and jazz—that is, when she's not busy earning As and Bs or working on Student Council or volunteering in a student program to educate freshmen about the dangers of drugs and the like. In the summers, she attends camps for Poms and dance. This is a girl with her head on straight.

Her body image varies depending on the type of activities she's doing and the time of the month. During her period, like the rest of us, she feels bloated and her tummy is "huge." When she's running from activity to activity, stretching, dancing, and cheering, she feels great about herself. Stick-thin celebrities, she said, do have an impact because they make her feel, "Why can't I be like that?" But she eats whatever and whenever she wants. She doesn't want to become overly obsessive about it.

Katie's favorite parts of her body are her legs. She could do without her butt, which is a bit too bootylicious for her taste, or her belly, which is fit but has "just a little pudge on the bottom." Her friend, let's call her Abby, has a fabulous stomach with rock-hard abs. That would be better.

Katie doesn't belong to a health club, but she has had ample locker room exposure nonetheless. Such as changing before gym class, or showering in communal showers during Poms competitions or summer camps (they wear bathing suits; remember those days when a shower just wasn't a shower if you weren't wearing a bathing suit?). She said that changing before gym class isn't a big deal for her. "I just change. I'm not like, 'Look at me,' but I just get it over with." Bras are kept on. As for underwear, for those girls who choose to wear thongs, they have adapted a changing technique even the most skillful of magicians would be jealous of: They stick their butts into the lockers as they pull their pants or skirts off so that nobody sees their bottoms. It reminds me of that classic trick where the magician "saws" the woman in the box in half. From the outside, everything appears neat and clean, but on the inside, it's a jumble of ruses and deceptions. The girls in the thongs appear to be confident and mature, but on the inside, they're scared and unsure of themselves, of their bodies. When Katie described this locker technique to me, it struck me as genius and absurd at the same time. I understand not wanting to moon the entire female contingent of your gym class, but then why wear a G-string to school? But then again, there's Amanda's whole Crabwalk philosophy. Maybe it's simply starting at a younger age.

I asked Katie whether a lot of teasing goes on in her locker room. She answered honestly and affirmatively, but only in response to "gross things," such as stretch marks or lack of cleanliness. But even then, the way she said it, I got the feeling she wasn't an active participant in the taunting. For instance, she described one girl who was overweight, but didn't openly call her "fat."

"She didn't really take care of herself," Katie said, and made a rather astute observation: "I don't think she was the happiest person." Katie also noticed what appeared to be self-inflicted cut marks on the girl's wrist. "I hope she went to see the school psychologist."

Two, Four, Six, Eight, Ads and Models Rule Our Fate!

Rana did me a huge favor by assembling a group of five high school ladies to meet at a café one Wednesday afternoon after school. All but one of them had come from cheerleading tryouts. I arrived and met a group of very cool and outspoken girls, all ages fifteen and sixteen: Rana, Emily, Fiona, Rhianna, and Meghan (some of whom I mentioned above). We squeezed into a booth and ordered (raspberry-peach smoothie for Rana; pineapple bubble tea for Emily; banana shake for Fiona; and a cookies 'n cream milkshake for Rhianna, which prompted giggles all around because Rhianna is biracial); Meghan, who arrived a bit later, didn't order.

As it turned out, these girls' insight into body image in general and what it's like contending with being a teenager in today's thin-is-in society was pure and incredibly perceptive. Even a simple question, such as "What's the first thing that pops into your head when I say the words 'body image'?" incited responses that I, the seasoned expert, wasn't expecting to hear.

For example, Rana, who seemed to assume the group's leadership role, began to speak of how, as a young ballerina, she miraculously managed to escape major body-image issues until the fifth grade when her teacher told her that if she "wanted to go anywhere" in ballet, she'd have to drop 10 pounds.

Rana described her body as small and compact but "not skinny," and said that last year, in an effort to become truly comfortable with her physique, she committed herself to working out regularly and building a buff body. During the summer, she can even attain a six-pack, and those lines of muscle in her stomach provide her with a deep sense of satisfaction.

But then—poof!—the satisfaction and acceptance seemed to disappear during cheerleading tryouts that afternoon when the other girls were unable to lift her. Although I'm not familiar with the ins and outs of cheerleading, this seemed odd to me, considering Rana looked as if I could easily hoist her onto my shoulder and carry her around with one arm. Her ego seemed more than slightly deflated when she recounted the story to all of us, as if not being able to be elevated into midair by a group of teenaged girls was something to ashamed of. (For the record, she made the team.)

Sixteen-year-old Emily had the *opposite* problem. Her natural thinness made her feel awkward, especially when it came to things like cheerleading tryouts, when her outfit hung in places it was meant to cling.

"In grade school, people used to pick me up and spin me and say, 'Emily, you're so skinny!'" she recounted. At this, all the other girls exchanged glances, their rolling eyes saying, "I *so* wanted to be that girl." (Fiona even later admitted, "When Emily was complaining about being skinny, I wanted to hit her. I would give anything to be skinny.") But not Emily. The constant taunting about her weight—or lack thereof—drove her to tears. To this day, she doesn't like it when people compliment her on almost anything.

Emily hasn't had many experiences in a health club locker room, although one in particular will forever remain with her. She was nine years old and her friend's mother had just undergone a breast reduction. Apparently they were still fairly large (or at least large in the eyes of a nine-year-old) because, as Emily put it, "I saw them in the locker room and I was like, 'Pow!' I haven't forgotten it. When you're little, you just want to be mature. I guess I just associated boobs with maturity." Perhaps that's why now, before gym class at school, she finds herself strategically maneuvering in the locker room so that no one will see her training bra.

The things about her body she does like? Her eyes, because they're "a weird color." She added, "I also like my nose, because it's big and Jewish."

Speaking of big and Jewish, Hollywood has had a definite impact on these girls' ideals of beauty and perfection (I'm Jewish, too, so it's okay if I make jokes like that). I spread out an array of magazine advertisements, some showing über-skinny models verging on the border of anorexia, others depicting full-figured models in lingerie. Rana took this chance to explain how images such as these alternately mold and shatter the body images of girls like them.

"TV shows say, 'This is perfection, this is what you're supposed to look like.' They take twenty-five-year-olds and put them in the roles of sixteen-year-olds." The result: Teenagers are presented with an unattainable ideal, an epitome of beauty they couldn't possibly achieve. And so—and this is just me playing armchair psychologist—they start getting Brazilian bikini waxes and wearing G-strings and having plastic surgery in a pathetic game of catch-up so that they can look like the girls on television and in the magazines.

One of the magazine ads I brought happened to have floated to the top, this one touting a cream for cellulite. I asked the ladies whether they think about such things as boob jobs and Botox and cellulite.

"What's cellulite?" Meghan asked in what was just about the most innocent and pure voice I have ever heard in my entire life.

Fuckfuckfuckfuckfuckfuck.

She looked into my eyes for an answer and I felt I'd been socked in the stomach—and rightfully so—for I may have just unwittingly dirtied one of the few unpolluted oceans remaining in Meghan's world. Oh, not to know what cellulite is! I thought toddlers today asked for Endermologie on their Christmas wish lists.

Rana stepped in and explained that cellulite is what happens when you do *this* (she attempted to grab excess flesh from her thigh and flank and push it together to achieve that wonderful orange-rind appearance but, alas, she was too well-toned.)

Meghan looked down at her long, beautiful legs, crossed at the knee, a horrified expression creeping across her face. "Do *I* have cellulite?" she asked me, grasping at her limbs. "No," I assured her. "You definitely don't have cellulite. You're beautiful." (Later, I would come to realize that what I had done, by my comments, was perpetuate the belief that one cannot be beautiful and have cellulite at the same time. There's one teachable moment down the tubes.) But still, it was enough to sooth body-image worries for the time being, and Meghan looked at me and smiled, her braces shining. Crisis averted . . . I hope.

To see whether I was on the right track regarding the media's impact on these young women, I consulted Karen Zager, PhD, a New York psychologist who works closely with young women and who wrote *The Inside Story on Teen Girls*. She said she hears the same thing from her teenaged clients. "The norm is to be very sexual," Dr. Zager said. "You don't have to have sex, but you have to be sexual—piercings, thongs, bikini waxes, weighing all of 62 pounds." And it's being pushed down to children of eleven and twelve: "They want to wear thongs, they want to get waxed—wax what?!"

Sabrena Newton, an exercise scientist with the American Council on Exercise, agreed that the images young women are exposed to, via popular magazines, can be detrimental to body image and self-worth. Newton, who has done fitness modeling, has been subjected to retouching and knows firsthand that even the most in-shape people are airbrushed and smoothed down. She stresses this to her teenaged clients, who bring in pictures from magazines, who complain about "how they hate their hips and thighs, how they jiggle." These girls are often barely sixteen years old.

On the positive side, Newton pointed out that mothers bringing their daughters to the health club does set a positive example about the importance of being fit—after all, it is called a *health* club. Nonetheless, that needs to be balanced, she said, by moms being "careful of what they expose their young daughters to and monitoring what they say about their [own] bodies."

She suggested mothers educate their daughters, perhaps by looking at magazines together and showing them how advertisements are altered. That way, Newton said, it's not quite as devastating, and they can understand they're comparing themselves to a fictitious representation of what a woman really looks like. "Let's face it," she said, "the media's not going away and I doubt if they're going to change anytime soon the way they represent models in magazines."

Giving Kids a Head Start on Self-Consciousness

We all know how early body-image concerns can begin to fester. In fact, my preschool teacher mother has actually had toddlers refuse cookies and juice because they were "on a diet." Yes. So I wanted to include some information about much younger girls. After all, like the three-year-old scale climber from Chapter 1, little ones scamper around my locker room all the time. Sometimes they seem oblivious to the nudity surrounding them, often admiring their bodies in the mirror as they dance around in their underwear or rake combs through each other's mousse-soaked hair. But at other times they seem quite conscious of where they are and what they're seeing. They'll stare, mouths agape, as women pull on thongs or straighten their hair, as heavyset women struggle with their bras or older women apply eye cream. You can literally see their view of what it means to be a woman being shaped before your very eyes.

I remember an occasion when a stereotypically beautiful woman (blonde hair, thin, made-up) was changing next to me. A mother rounded the corner carrying her baby and the baby smiled, pointed at the blonde, and said "Pwitty." Even at such a young age, the infant recognized conventionally accepted beauty and associated being blonde with big eyes and red lips with something positive. More recently, a young girl mistook a well-toned black woman wearing sweats and a bandana around her forehead for a man as we were all lined up at the makeup counter. I later saw that woman naked in the steam room, long hair spread out around her head and a gorgeous face, and I kid you not when I say her body rivaled that of Halle Berry. It just goes to show what young girls are conditioned to think of as feminine and attractive, and how early that conditioning happens.

Another experience that sticks out in my mind occurred when I had a suspicious mole removed from beneath my left breast and the dermatologist prescribed a special ointment for me to apply to help prevent scarring. However, to apply the gel properly, I needed to use my left hand to lift up my breast while I rubbed the gel over the wound.

One afternoon, as I stood at the mirror, breast in hand, towel wrapped around my waist, four little girls no more than five years old walked in and caught sight of me. Like ducks in a row, they passed by, each one giggling as she looked first at me and then at her friends in the mirror, hands over mouths. I could almost *see* the thoughts rising over their heads: "That lady's touching her boob!"

To help me gather more insight, I enlisted Dawn Penney, a registered dance therapist and licensed professional counselor who manages a children's club associated with a gym here in Chicago. Penney, who herself battled anorexia and bulimia for more than a decade, gets along fabulously with children; she speaks their language, whereas my conversation skills with those under the age of ten is limited to "Hiiii-eee!" (The other day at a friend's party, I actually asked a five-year-old with a sore throat whether she wanted some hot tea.) But Penney was handily able to gather a group of girls ranging from three and a half to seven for a ballet movement class and, with their parents' permission, they gathered to practice their dance skills and answer our body-related questions.

The answers began as inspiring insight into self-image and body awareness. For example, when Penney sat everyone in a circle and asked what their favorite body part was, poignant answers flooded in such as "My heart, because I love my mommy and daddy," from Annika; "My eyes, because I can see my favorite things," from Carly; and "My nose, because I can smell my favorite things," from Payton. Olivia, the youngest, wandered away to admire herself in her pink tutu. So far, so good.

"What about your legs?" Miss Dawn asked, a question that would normally inspire riots among grown women as they fought to shout their dislikes over one another. (I, for instance, have cankle issues.) "They help us walk!" was the consensus. Huh. No talk of chubby thighs or ankles. How refreshing. Everything was sweet and inspiring so far. In fact, the only negative reaction to a body part Penney could elicit had to do with a little girl's hair being pulled into a too-tight bun.

But when the conversation started to incorporate words such as "fat" and "skinny," it quickly devolved into a sad commentary on body image and today's little girl:

PENNEY: "Who has heard the word 'fat'?"
EVERYONE: "Me!"

PENNEY: "Is it okay to be fat?"
COLLECTIVE: "No!"
CARLY: "Because you'd probably break things and be sad."

Here's where it started to go downhill . . .

PENNEY: "Do you think you'd have friends if you were fat?"
COLLECTIVE: "No!"

PENNEY: "Do you think people who are fat are happy?"
COLLECTIVE: "No!"

PENNEY: "Do you think people who are fat are smart?"
COLLECTIVE: "No!"

PENNEY: "What does it mean to be skinny?"

This was difficult for them to conceptualize, so Penney rephrased, "Is it better to be skinny or fat?"

COLLECTIVE: "Skinny!"

PENNEY: "Would you have friends if you were skinny?"
Collective: "Yes!"

PENNEY: "Would you be smart if you were skinny?"
COLLECTIVE: "Yes!"

At this point Penney looked at me and whispered, "I feel like crying."

PENNEY: "Who told you it's better to be skinny than fat?"
THREE GIRLS REPLIED: "Mommy and Daddy."

PENNEY: "What do you think when you see people in the locker room next door?"

My head was reeling so much that I didn't catch who called out, "It's really funny to see people without clothes!" but by that time it was practically a moot point.

It's true that these children may have just been practicing herd mentality by all replying with the same answer. And sure, they might be blaming "Mommy and Daddy" simply because they're not old enough to understand or recognize external factors such as peer pressure or the media. (After all, when asked, "Has anyone ever heard the word 'diet'?" Julia's immediate response was "Diet Coke!" These kids are bombarded with diet-conscious ads.) But the sad bottom line is, even at such young ages, little girls already associate being fat with being dumb, friendless, and even dangerous (well, to furniture, anyway). How long before babies begin requesting skimmed breast milk and asking one another, "Does this diaper make my butt look big?" And they're learning it from us.

But a few weeks later, a sliver of hope emerged on the horizon: As I made my way up the staircase to the locker room at my gym, I was forced to stop as a gaggle of little kids and their parents spilled past me like some crazy human avalanche. Mixed in with all the screaming and parental pleading to move faster, I heard a little girl, maybe seven years old, cry out, "But I don't *want* carrots for dinner! I want a real meal!" Keep shouting, baby. Maybe there's hope for you yet.

12

Having a Senior Moment

What Lessons Can the Older Generation Teach Us?

In the course of my gym-going exploits, I've been exposed to many older women in the locker room. And when I say exposed, I really mean *exposed*. Not in a bad way. Older women, in my experience, tend to have shed their self-consciousness with age and I try to let their freedom rub off on me, or at least sink in via osmosis. Like caterpillars having spent their fair share of time working away in the cocoon of life, going through so many experiences and transitions, these mature women have finally emerged. Contrary to popular thought, *they* are the butterflies of the locker room, not the young ladies flitting about in their low-slung gym shorts and shrunken sorority baby tees. It just so happens that typically, when one "emerges" from any sort of womb, insect or human, she tends to be naked. And older women . . . well, in the locker room, they just always seem to be naked. And confident to boot.

Why shouldn't they? They have given birth and survived illness and disease. They have outlived husbands and, in some cases, children. They fought for equal rights in work and education. These women have accumulated more wisdom and knowledge in their salon-styled hairdos than we have in our entire, body-image-obsessed, toned-to-the-hilt selves. Typically, barring the ones who, after decades of struggle, continue to battle eating issues, they have boatloads to offer us in the way of lessons of self-acceptance. And even the ones who still struggle have lessons to teach us.

I often hear women of my age complain about "the old ladies in my gym who walk around completely naked with their boobs down by their waists and their stomachs hanging out." Then they add, "I don't want to see that." Well, guess what, gals? Like it or not, you're looking into a very powerful mirror. So I'll take the wrinkles. And the knowledge. Any day.

Now, this is not to say that all the older women in my locker room—or yours, for that matter—are wrinkled and drooping. Some have great genes, some have never given birth, some have had plastic surgery, or Botox, or both. And some just work their asses off, plain and simple, to win the war against gravity. But regardless of whether their bodies look like maps or SAPs (Senior American Princesses), I have never seen a woman of sixty or older scurry off into a bathroom stall to change or quickly scan the room before dropping her towel and pulling on her underwear . . . be it granny-style or G-string.

One of my earliest memories of interacting with senior-aged women in the locker women happened more than a decade ago. After working out and showering at my suburban gym, I was rushing to get dressed. Bra clasped, shirt pulled over wet hair, and jeans yanked on, I grabbed my socks from my locker and supported my weight on my bent right leg. I lifted my left knee to my chest, reverse pelican-style, so I could slip my left foot in first. Apparently, a group of women—I'm guessing they were in their sixties or seventies—donning swimsuits and caps, had been watching me.

"Look at that," one said to another, knowing full well I could hear their conversation. "Remember when we could do that?"

"Oy, such balance," she replied, smiling in only the way an older person recounting memories of her youth can. Then, addressing me directly, one commented, "We used to be able to put our socks on like you, rushing around in such a hurry. Not anymore."

For some reason, I recall that conversation with arctic clarity. Maybe I was having an Oprah "Aha!" moment (even though this was before they existed). I just remember knowing something important had transpired. An intergenerational life lesson. Of course, at the time I was a silly teenager, more concerned with rushing off to whatever party or hang-out session I was planning to attend. But subconsciously, it hit me. Not to take basic skills, such as balance, for granted. Years later, when my mom was diagnosed with multiple sclerosis, that lesson came back to help me understand her trials and tribulations.

Eve Ensler of *The Vagina Monologues* fame wrote a short tome called *The Good Body* that was centered around her hatred of her once-flat but now rounded belly. In it, she interviews a seventy-four-year-old African Masai woman named Leah about her body image. When Ensler asks Leah whether she likes her body, she points to a tree and says, "Eve, look at that tree? Do you see that tree? Now look at *that* tree. Do you like that tree? Do you hate that tree 'cause it doesn't look like that tree?"

Leah continues, "We're all trees. You're a tree. I'm a tree. You've got to love your body, Eve. You've got to love your tree."

Here is what real older women shared with me about their body images and how they've come to love their bodies and their selves (for those who have, that is)—from a fifty-eight-year-old former ballerina to a ninety-one-year-old yoga instructor. They say with age comes wisdom. Time to smarten up.

Shelly, seventy-four, a retired teacher and travel agent:

"You should hear us after class in the swimmer's locker room. Just this morning the girls and I were having a conversation—one woman's husband had had a stroke, one had cancer of the colon, one said he was depressed and he was on antidepressants and you know what I did? I looked at her and I said, 'You need to be on one, too.' We all laughed, but it's true. I think . . . women are finally realizing they can talk to other women. Women in my age group never had other women to talk to. If you were depressed after you had a baby, you just didn't talk about it. And we're learning from the younger women. Even though what they talk about are things like arranging play dates for their kids, they *talk*.

"Do we care about being naked in front of each other? Nooo. The women in my age group—we sort of look at each other and laugh. You know, 'When did they drop?' They used to be perky and all of the sudden they're down by our waists. And the younger women, it's interesting. They listen. I don't know if they think we're a bunch of nuts or what. We laugh, we're very assertive. I'll look at myself in the mirror and say, 'When did my thighs start to look like this?'

"My workout is usually low-impact, stretching and water classes. I have a very bad back, so it's limiting me. Plus, I have arthritis and a bulging disk. It's wonderful stuff. So I work around it. I'm comfortable with my body. You reach an age where you realize this is it—it's not going to change. Accept yourself and love yourself for what you are and don't let anyone else tell you what to be.

"I'll look at some of the young, gorgeous women in the locker room and I'll tease them. I'll say, 'You're not allowed in this part of the locker room,' or 'Put a big paper bag over everything!' They're flattered. Because they're darling and they should be proud of it. You're all tall, and you're all slender and you're all beautiful."

June, sixty-nine, the executive vice president of a fitness education company:

"If you will allow me to be immodest, I'm sixty-nine and look as though I'm forty-five. My boyfriend is six years younger than I am and my daughter and I share the same clothes. It's wonderful feeling this way at my age.

"I work out a minimum of four times a week. I'll do the cross trainer and hike on the weekends for at least an hour and a half, and then I do extensive weight training with a trainer three times per week. My daughter owns a yoga company and I teach classes there, too.

"As a young girl growing up in a rural country area of New Jersey, I was definitely athletic. Always on the go—I don't sit well. There was no television, so we were always outside doing something. In my twenties and thirties, I didn't go to a gym but I did a lot of walking—living in New York

City, I walked at least three miles a day. My ex-husband and I had a boat and we'd go swimming in the summertime.

"Yes, body image was a concern. I was totally flat-chested—two raisins on a breadboard, I used to call myself. So I got implants at forty-three, when my husband and I divorced. I was single again and wanted a little something. I didn't go huge, just a 34B. They made me feel much sexier.

"In my early forties, I started running and joined a gym. We did aerobics. But the real changes came with yoga. Yoga changed my body more than anything. It made me very strong, especially in my upper body.

"I get dressed in my office before I head to the gym, so I don't need to use the locker room. But in the locker room I used to use, I was in my forties at that time, a lot of the girls were younger than myself. I got hit on a couple of times—living in New York City, I was a street-savvy woman and I just knew that's what was happening. It didn't bother me that much. I just didn't respond. They got the hint.

"Speaking of getting hit on, I feel very sensual at this age, more sensual than at any other age. But I think it has to do with the man and his response. My boyfriend is very positive about my physique—he looks at me and says I have the body of a twenty-five-year-old. I mean, not really—I have wrinkles and sagging skin, but I work at it. When I was forty-five, I was still wearing a string bikini and I definitely wouldn't do that today, but I do feel good in my skin. You have to be happy with yourself inside before you can have any kind of decent relationship.

"Now my daughter, her body is incredible. She's thirty-nine years old and very tall. Growing up, I always reminded her to stand up straight, because there's nothing worse than slouching shoulders. It's very regal to stand up straight. She never developed breasts so she got implants like me, too. She credits me with her initiation into working out. When I started to exercise, she was in high school and says I set a good example. So that makes me feel very good."

Harriet, fifty-seven, a public relations executive:

"I am fifty-seven and work out about three to four times per week. Body image has been an ongoing thorn in my side since way before puberty. Since I always considered myself 'fat,' working out has been an obsession for nearly forty-seven years.

"Some kids used to say I had piano legs. Back in those days, girls weighed 110, 115. I was 125. But I was flexible— I could do backbends, stretches. Unfortunately, from those stupid comments, I saw myself as being very fat. Still do.

"I started working out in junior high. I was active in sports. At sixteen, I started swimming laps three times a week. I kept that up until I was fifty. My husband knew that if I didn't get my exercise routine in, I would be a menace to live with. The problem was, I never saw a change in my body. After a while, I'd add more on, like I would Rollerblade two miles to the pool, swim laps, and then Rollerblade home. Still, nothing. But now that I'm in my fifties, I've come to realize it kept my body aerobically toned and in good health. Now I do the elliptical, lift weights, and yoga—that's made a big change. I started yoga four years ago. My muscles are more sculpted. People say I look like I've lost weight, but I haven't. I'm just more toned. Oh, and I follow a low-carb diet. So I guess you could say I started working out for vanity, but now the motivators have changed to both vanity and health. So I got to the same place for different reasons, but I am thankful I am here, nonetheless. Had I not worked out as much as I did through-out my life, I might be like other fifty-seven-year-olds with myriad health problems. Instead, I have never been to a hospital except for childbirth and I have the flexibility and stamina I had as a teen.

"One of my daughters is actually significantly overweight and it terrifies me. Not obese, but still. She used to be a stunningly beautiful girl when she lived in my house. I didn't allow fast food and I made them exercise. But as soon as she went to college, all my efforts went down the drain. So now we're doing Weight Watchers together.

"Right now, I'm thinking of getting a face-lift, but you can't work out for four weeks afterward and that terrifies me. Actually, anytime there has been a threat of gaining weight, I become anxious. Like during pregnancy; I gained 45 pounds with each pregnancy, even though I worked out every day with both kids. Or if my husband wants to take me on a cruise; everyone knows you gain weight on a cruise. I guess you could say the possibility of getting bigger has been the primary motivator behind a lot of my choices in my life.

"So back to the face-lift. I have a sagging chin and my eyes are going down. My husband says they make me look sad. And I'm not—I'm upbeat, I'm blessed to have two great kids, I love my job, my health is excellent. I exercise, so I've got the endorphins running around. The only thing holding me back is a lack of time off from my job and the exercise issue.

"Now as an empty-nester, I have more time to work out. And I like it. I really enjoy it. I even taught myself to speak Indonesian on the elliptical machine. And I am the oldest person in my Ashtanga yoga class by decades. I can do head stands, push ups, all of it.

"I won't leave the gym without showering. I have to get clean. But in the locker room, my least favorite part is blow-drying my hair. It's just so boring. You want to go home, you're hungry from working out and want to eat. I hate it.

"No, I'm not modest—I'll strip in front of anybody. One of the things age has done is made me totally not modest about my body. I walk around my house nude, too. Maybe it comes from growing up in the late 1960s. But once I got married, I wasn't hung up about showing my body anymore, even though at 145, I'm about 20 pounds more than I weighed throughout high school. When I was younger—before fifty, ha ha—I was still more self-conscious about my body because I thought I had fat legs. Now, I am more comfortable with my body, even with the weight.

"Looking back, the thought that I was obese at 125 pounds makes me laugh. Why did I think I was obese? My youngest daughter weighs a couple of pounds more than I did and we're the same height and she has the most beautiful figure. I mean, she's put together a little differently: Her weight is mostly in the bust and she has a slimmer legs and hips. But I still marvel at that. Sometimes I look at this picture of myself as a young girl and think, wow, I based so many decisions in my life on the fear of gaining weight."

Paula, seventy-two, a mother and grandmother:

"Exercise wasn't always a part of my life. I've been working out about thirty years. My husband was the impetus. He lost his whole family to coronary artery disease—his brothers, his father, his mother. So he started exercising and it changed our whole life. He was getting up at six in the morning, going to the YMCA and running, so I thought I'd see what it was all about, beginning in my early forties. I enjoyed it . . . after a while (laughs). It wasn't because it changed my body or for the health benefits. I had five children and I could just head out my front door and think and be alone and be quiet and that's what I liked the best.

"Before I had children, I was thinner. I had a little waist. We used to wear Merry Widows. But you change. And as a matter of fact, I have a daughter with four children and I asked her, 'Why aren't you all wrinkled up?' Of course, exercise was not acceptable when I was pregnant. You were supposed to sit on the couch and eat bon-bons.

"I've been on a diet my whole life, on every diet ever invented. You name it, I've been on it. That was a part of our life when we were young, unless you were a really skinny person. The pressure was everywhere. It's not the same kind of pressure as young girls feel now, because now they want to be disgusting looking. You didn't make yourself sick like people do today. But you were on that chalky Metrecal or whatever it was.

"Now I'm on Weight Watchers, even though I'm not overweight. It's for maintenance. One of my daughters and I do it together. But I also think it's important to watch what you eat because of your health, to keep your cholesterol down, all of that stuff. And I go to the gym pretty regularly. I'll do the treadmill or elliptical, Step classes, weight training classes, and Spinning.

"I've been lucky to have met a wonderful group of women in the locker room at my gym. There's a definite camaraderie in the locker room. We change together. We go to lunch. I know about their children, who's getting aggravated by what, pictures of the grandchildren and all of that. We've become friends. One of the girls spends six weeks in Mexico every year and my husband and I go down and visit her—and she and I met in the locker room!

"Most of the women my age cover up in the locker room. And chunky ladies cover, young or old. But let me tell you, I still remember this story and it still makes me angry: When I was younger, I used to run the swimming club at my high school and the gym teacher would make us girls take our swimsuits off to shower and then we had to walk naked to get our stuff. Now, I thought that was awful—I still think that's terrible. If a girl wants to cover herself up, she should be able to. The young girls in the club today, they walk around naked in the locker room. It doesn't offend me. They're beautiful, so why not?

"And my body, what can I say about my body? It's mine. I tease about it and say, 'Uch, it's not a pretty sight.' You've got gravity. It's not like those pretty young things. But it's mine."

Patty, fifty-eight, a lawyer, former ballerina:

"I started studying ballet when I was younger than five and the belief was, the thinner your were, the more value you had. We learned how not to eat and we did it because we wanted to be the prima ballerina. The older girls taught each other how to purge or be anorexic. It was a secret society.

"For me, the eating stuff began when I was nine or ten and started dancing on pointe shoes. You wanted to be the star. I danced until I was forty-seven, keeping active with lessons and in companies. The actual eating disorder didn't stay that long, but I've always had eating issues, and I've always been able to spot them. I remember in my thirties, one of the dance companies had hired a new dancer, and during a performance, she started shaking. My husband and I were in the audience and I leaned over and whispered 'That's an amphetamine shake.' He asked, 'Well, how do you know?' It's because I took them. At the time we called them diet pills. The physicians prescribed them to us. I was five foot two, weighed 90 pounds soaking wet, and thought I was fat.

"In my early forties, I started to notice that I was getting tired a lot, gaining weight around my middle, where you used to be able to feel my pelvic bones. I was losing my hair. As it turned out, I had Cushings, which is a tumor on the adrenal gland that pumps out steroids. My blood pressure was sky-high, I had ballooned from a size 1 to a 12, and I was a raging diabetic. I felt grotesque-looking. People on the street would make these 'Tsk' noises. Everything I believed in my youth came true—if you're not thin, you have no value. If you can't control your weight, you have no value.

"I had surgery to remove the tumor, and it was as if somebody put a pin in me and the weight just came off. But along with it, a little bit of my eating-disorder mentality returned, so I had to keep that in check. Even now, at 105 pounds, I wear a size 2, sometimes a 4, and the littlest bit of change makes me wonder—am I getting fat? That's hard for me to admit.

"I try to eat very sensibly. I will never put donuts in my mouth. Maybe I'm afraid the Cushings will come back. Maybe it's the thought of being overweight—I don't think it will ever end for me. I want to be healthy, but I don't think it will be 'healthy' in the medical profession sense . . . 'healthy' will always be too fat for me.

"My daughter knows about my past. I felt if I hid it from her, it would be disastrous. I wanted her to know that when we danced, it wasn't the best culture for body image. And I am able to look at other women who aren't stick thin and appreciate their beauty. So how come I can't be happy with myself? So I've always tried to instill lessons in my daughter like make sure you have good girlfriends for support, make sure you have people you trust, and always have someone to tell you that you look gorgeous."

ArLyne, sixty-nine, a corporate consultant, former therapist:

"I guess you could say I was a late bloomer. When I was a teenager, my closest friend had a real Marilyn Monroe shape. Not me. I used to joke that the boys would ask me to carry their books so they could carry hers. But when I got into my early twenties, I started to model professionally. I was a dressmaker dummy in New York, and then I also had occasion to see myself on video, like when I stood up as maid of honor at a girlfriend's wedding. Seeing myself objectively, I realized I had a great figure. So I came into my own wonderfully.

"Aging from twenty to thirty helped me to love my body more and then in my thirties and forties, I was in a great relationship—your body image is always good when you're in a great relationship. But aging from fifty to sixty-nine didn't help at all. I was involved in two auto accidents in the late 1980s and gained 50 pounds. I went from having a beautiful figure to becoming an apple—and seeing my mother when I look in the mirror. Plus, I was diagnosed with diabetes.

"But my critical damage point was my hair. All my life I had gorgeous red hair. I mean, beautiful, all natural, stop-traffic red hair. And as I got older, that changed. That was a bigger issue for me than my weight.

"All of this affected me somewhat, emotionally. Obviously, it was disappointing—I wasn't initially comfortable with the weight, but I didn't go into hiding because of it. I don't really have a sense of myself being overweight. I dress exceptionally well and don't try to be somebody I'm not. What I know is that it's how you feel that matters—not how you look. When you feel good about yourself, you're not as critical about your body image.

"I work out fairly erratically. Some light weight training, ballroom dancing, walking. I used to do kung fu, but they closed my dojo. So I'm not in locker rooms too often. When I am, I can say I'm not at all modest. It goes back to my modeling days. I'm comfortable in my own person. I like me. And consequently, the fact that my body isn't what I want isn't that big of a deal. I might compare myself to other women: Is my butt as big as her butt? I notice the young, really nubile women. But it doesn't elevate to hazardous levels. Just momentary flashes of discontent.

"When I was a kid, I remember going to a resort with my family. I was in a steam bath and I haven't thought about this for so long, but it was really frightening to see these women with big breasts who had lost all of their firmness. Seeing that image as a child frightened me. To me, it represented women being dried out and wasted and I don't feel that way about myself at all. And I have always had gorgeous breasts. I've always been able to go without a bra. Well, until now.

"I think we put an enormous amount of horrible, ugly pressure on women to meet some unattainable standard. It's always been there: first Marilyn Monroe, then Twiggy, then Britney Spears. As a therapist, it was so awful to see women view themselves as falling short. I'd be horrified when someone would come in and say, 'My husband told me my thighs were too big during sex.' That is so, so destructive, a comment like that coming from a man who professes to love you.

"Oh, I've got an interesting story. Years ago, one of my clients was a concert pianist, and she had a shortened thumb. She was adorable, a cute woman with a darling figure, but every room she walked into, she would judge her thumb against other peoples' thumbs. That became the yardstick against which she measured herself. Her thumb was our weight.

"As I've grown older, there is less of a sense of body image and more of a sense of a loss of image, if you know what I mean. I conduct workshops on aging and one of the things I can tell you is more than body image, many older women are starting to feel invisible. That has a profound impact on women. Men my age still notice me, but there aren't that many men my age! And to young men, I'm just an old woman. You don't get that acknowledgment. Still, I think I am very attractive, for my age. Men, on the other hand, age more gracefully than women. In today's society, it's far more acceptable to be an older man, which pisses me off, frankly."

Linda, sixty-three, an author and psychotherapist:

"As a young girl, I was always embarrassed because I was the tallest girl in class, with ugly toes. My mother rejected me, saying I was plain looking. People would tell me I was a beautiful girl and I thought they were lying to me. Looking back now, I can see it was a competition sort of thing. She was competing with me. I didn't actually feel pretty until my 30s. When I grew older and looked back at pictures, I asked, 'Holy cow, why couldn't I enjoy that beauty?'

"I developed anorexia in my teens. At five foot eight, I dropped down to 128, when I usually weighed 140. Now that scared my mom. She couldn't make me eat. Later on in life, as a psychotherapist, I treated anorexic girls. I think what I was doing was trying to get her to see that my life was in danger from our relationship, how her lack of love was affecting me. That's why it's been so important for me to be a good mother to myself.

"Today, at sixty-three, I am a post-polio survivor. I originally contracted polio at age eleven and couldn't walk. My throat was paralyzed and I couldn't eat, speak, or breathe on my own for a while . . . a year I think.

"Then, in my early fifties, I awoke one day to bone-crushing fatigue and swallowing troubles. It was post-polio syndrome, and it left me with severe arthritis. I knew I had to build a loving relationship with my body—which I did—and that has had a powerful effect on my healing.

"I remember a friend said to me, 'You never had good mothering. Now it's time to be a mother to yourself.' So every morning I say things to myself like, 'What do you need today?'

"I also use other methods to nurture my body, such as restorative yoga, resting my neck every day, and traveling to exotic places with my husband, where we snorkel. I stay hydrated. I pray. I treat my body as I would treat someone I love very much. These acts have brought me to radiant and resilient health—so much so that I have gone from crippling joint pain to being pain-free, without medication.

"A lot of women carry shame about how we look. Many of us are undergoing surgery, even at a very young age. One of my tips is to massage every part of the body with scented oil and a brush. As I do this, I thank each part of my body. My feet for their steadfastness. My legs for their beauty and strength. My stomach for my creativity. My back for my responsibility. It's very affirming and gets rid of so much negativity about our body image.

"I now have a totally different relationship with my body—a very loving relationship. I feel beautiful. I am my body's loving mother. I am dancing again, no longer using a cane, and am told that I look younger now than I did ten years ago. I have transformed my inner critic to an approver who can appreciate my body's strength. I don't even go to the gym because I don't want to leave my beautiful home to do a regimented routine. Sometimes I'll walk or swim. Or maybe I'll just put on 'Earth, Wind and Fire' and I boogie."

Sandy "Dr. Sandy" Goldberg, sixty, a clinical nutritionist and television health and nutrition contributor:

"Body image has been so intertwined with my life, I don't ever remember *not* being aware of it. I was an obese child, so it was something I dealt with constantly. My parents tried absolutely everything. I remember at age six, being excused at 11:00 a.m. from class to take a pill—subsequently, I learned these were diet pills. I went to spas, camps, lectures, the whole bit. Back then, exercise was not at the forefront like it is now. I was probably just eating too much.

"The major change came when I was twenty-six. I lost 160 pounds . . . and have kept it off for thirty-two years! I guess the straw that broke the camel's back was one morning, I reached over to tie my shoe and I couldn't—my stomach got in the way, my breasts got in the way. I mean, I was five foot three and weighed 280 pounds. Then I tried lifting my leg up onto a chair and I couldn't even do that. So I decided, that's it. I'm never going to feel this way again. I joined Weight Watchers and lost 125 pounds. Up to that point, I had probably lost and gained 2,000 pounds with yo-yo dieting. But I'm the kind of person who, once I decide to do something, I do it. And that morning, I decided.

"Then, I became very interested in food and went back to school. I already had a master's in comparative literature, but that wasn't going to help me get where I wanted to go, so I earned my master's and PhD, both in clinical nutrition. I believe the education, combined with the empathy I possessed, having lived as an overweight person, gave me a big edge. You understand your client. There's a bond. Plus, I had been bulimic. But back then, there was no term for it.

"I basically divide my life into Before the weight loss and After. Before, when I walked down the street, I was always the biggest person. People would stare at me. So I would try to make myself as anonymous as I could, which was virtually impossible. But losing weight . . . physically, it was a lot of fun to watch myself get smaller. And now, because of my affiliation with NBC, I'd like to think that when people stare, it's for a different reason.

"Do I love my body? It's almost unrealistic to say you love your body because most of us have parts of our bodies we don't love and never will. I still have some baggage. I think it's important to accept that we are who we are, but it's our responsibility to give ourselves the best shot at learning how to be comfortable with our body—eating properly, getting movement, not smoking. I walk everyday—I don't go to the gym. Movement is very important for the heart, lungs, but it has to work for you.

"Remember, your best friend and worst enemy is the person you see in the mirror. Stop being in a contest with yourself. Do what you have to do and don't expect overnight success, because there is no such animal."

Elaine, sixty-nine, author:

"I really can't say that I have a problem with the way my body looks. I had a mastectomy at forty-four, my gall bladder out, my appendix out, so I have many scars, but scars don't bother me. I've always said if my head was missing, my wonderful husband could still identify me—and he wears bifocals! Maybe I don't look like I did when I was twenty-one but I'm smarter than I was when I was twenty-one and that's what matters: what's in your head, your heart, your soul.

"The first time body image really entered my life was when I was ten years old. My family was at the lake in northwestern Iowa and I had rheumatic fever. The doctor came to visit and he had me take my shirt off, run up and down to the lake, and then checked my heart. I'm not sure why he had me take off my shirt. Then, when I was twelve or thirteen, I was a tomboy, and I wore overalls with a T-shirt but no bra a lot and I remember my older sister telling my mother I wasn't wearing a bra. That same older sister wound up struggling with anorexia and bulimia in middle age and, sadly, it wound up contributing to her death.

"As for me, I'm not a mirror person. I can look in the mirror at 3:00 P.M. and realize I've been wearing one earring all day. I belong to a health club and I'm fairly modest—I don't parade to the toilet without any clothes on, but I don't go to great lengths to hide my mastectomy scars, either. Nobody's ever commented on them. And I have spider veins, too, but you know what? The body is just a casing. I remember sitting with a bunch of women and they were asking each other, 'What part of your body do you hate?' This was just a few years ago. I didn't participate because I thought, 'How sad to hate any part of yourself . . . and what message does that send to our children?' I've got a seven-year-old granddaughter who asks me, 'Grandma, is this the healthy bread?' And I say, 'Yes, it is, but we can put some peanut butter on it because even though it has fat in it, it's good for you and you need to grow.' It's starting so young.

"I walk three miles, four times a week, and I lift weights. I want to stay healthy—that's the goal. Losing my breast was not a big deal; I was more afraid of the cancer. That's what scared the hell out of me. I wanted to see my ten-year-old grow up. I've tried to lower the stress in my life and I stay away from toxic people. I'm comfortable with my body image because it hasn't changed—reality has! It's harder to find clothes today because I'm short—just four foot eleven—and I can't buy in the children's department anymore. In my mind, I'm still the under-100-pound-girl with the pixie haircut. Well, at least I still have the haircut, but the scale has crept up. Who cares? I'm happy."

Kooki, sixty-seven, the owner of a company that plans senior outings:

"In my thirties, I became a borderline anorexic. I'd been heavy as a child and didn't know how to lose the weight. But then I had a hysterectomy and while I was in the hospital, I lost a lot of weight. I was thrilled, and I tried keeping it off. It got to the point where I weighed 79 pounds—I was five foot one at the time; right now I'm a little under five feet tall. My doctor did say he would like me to put on some weight, but I thought he was crazy; I was very happy being slender.

"The problem stayed with me for a long while. When my husband died thirteen years ago, I started eating a little more. I met someone special a while ago, which helped, but I still am very careful to eat healthfully. Now, I'd say I love myself but I'm happy being slender. It's not an obsession but a healthy awareness. I'm happy with my body. I guess my favorite part would have to be my rear!

"I have two daughters and a son, and I talked with my girls a lot about body image. Unfortunately, one of them became severely anorexic at around twelve or thirteen. She's forty-six now and still not doing well. She exercises like a fiend. It's a terrible disease because it doesn't leave you—it's always behind your head. The other one is overly concerned but has been successful in avoiding the disease because she's seen how destructive it can be. But the pressure is so bad—she has daughters and I hear my granddaughter say, 'I'm so fat, I'm so fat.' She and her friends comment on each other's bodies. They're sixteen. At least at the gym I see girls getting very strong. That seems to be more important to them than their weight, which is great.

"Now I'm at the gym three to five days a week. I prefer the classes, like Step and body sculpting. I also do Pilates one-on-one every other week and have physical therapy for spinal arthritis. In the locker room, even though we might not all be the same age, we all have similar interests. We're concerned about health. A lot of us are Jewish, so we discuss the holidays or things that affect Jewish women. We've all been friends for twenty years, so we're very concerned about each other. You know, if someone doesn't show up. That's a very nice, comforting thing to have."

Pat Brown, sixty-four, the president of the American Association for Nude Recreation:

"My jump into nudism was not a jump so much as it was a slow crawl. I joined in 1983 with my husband—he wanted to go to a clothing-optional beach. We're best friends and it was important to him. For me, I had to accept that my body was not the sum and substance of who I was before I could truly enjoy it. Which is something I think is especially difficult for women—we are taught from a very young age that our bodies are what matter. But once I realized how comfortable it was to be clothes-free, and when I was able to say my body didn't dictate who I was, it gave me a confidence—a confidence in my *nude* body even—that I'd never had before.

"Because of that, being in the locker room has never been a problem. But I remember one time, a woman said to me, 'Oh, do you feel like you're better than everyone else?' because I was walking around in the nude. It's a locker room! And the AARN's mission statement is 'Nude in appropriate places.' What's more appropriate than a ladies' locker room? But everyone has a different level of tolerance. So when she said that to me, my initial reaction was that of surprise; I wasn't flaunting anything. Rather, I was feeling so comfortable in the fact that I didn't have to look better than anyone else. I apologized and explained I had no intention of offending anyone. 'This is just the body I was born in,' I said. But then *she* apologized to *me*, saying it was a rather brusque comment she had made.

"I would not call my body a beautiful body. I'm sixty-four. I've had three kids. I have sagging skin from losing a lot of weight at one point, and I had a breast reduction. But I feel comfortable in it because I feel it's representative of bodies everywhere and after all, my body isn't *Pat*. Pat is what's inside. It's like my husband says, it's the only one I have and I've got lots of other things to do with my life other than obsess about a perfect body. Like when I'm out in the garden, working in the nude—I feel at one with the earth. I feel a part of that garden. We have an outdoor shower and I love it for the same reason—it is so wonderful to shower beneath the trees with no walls, like being in a waterfall. At those moments, what my body looks like . . . I don't want to say I'm oblivious because I'm healthy, I exercise, I follow a healthy diet, but it's not all that's on my mind."

Donna, fifty-six, a preschool teacher, author's mom:
"I was thirteen when I began what would turn out to be a lifetime of body-image issues. First it was scoliosis; I had to wear a 25-pound body cast from my chin to my hips to prevent surgery. It was horrible. The doctor outfitted me with these special glasses because my head faced upward with the cast, so when you looked upward into the glasses, you actually saw what was directly in front of you. So that was one of my first physical roadblocks. I wore that thing eight months on, six months off, eight months on again. Boys called me names. My physical education teacher gave me an F because I couldn't participate in tumbling or get on the balance beam. Can you believe that? I still remember her name. How sad that someone who was given responsibility in helping form a young woman's self-image was so insensitive.

"Then there was the high school locker room. I hated it. I remember I wasn't fully matured like some of the other girls, so getting undressed was unpleasant. That and showering. In fact, I remember the only way we could get out of showering was if we had our period. And I was a late bloomer, so I didn't get my period until I was fifteen. But I was embarrassed, so I made up a schedule, and every month, I had my 'period' and got out of showering in the locker room for a week. But then, I got it for real. And my teacher yelled at me, 'Donna, you just had it last week!'

"Oy, it's been a mess. I've got scars from surgery I had at birth so I was never able to wear tank tops. Just another, 'Oh well.' But I still dated, still went to dances. I tried to never let it get in the way of my social life. And in fact, I was a pretty girl. In college, I had long, straight hair to my waist. I wore go-go boots and minidresses and felt very good about myself, didn't feel the need to join a sorority.

"Pregnancy? I loved being pregnant. It was the first time I had breasts! My husband and I were going to bronze my bra. But then, I almost died giving birth to both of my children. Oh, but the tradeoff was worth it.

"When Leslie was growing up, she had a thyroid problem, which both her grandmother and I have. I realized body image was becoming more and more important. And as she gained weight as a younger girl and each symptom popped up—the dry skin, being cold all the time, the fatigue—it wasn't until I started playing detective and acted as an advocate for my daughter, that I got the doctors to really listen. And she got her medicine and the weight came off and she shot up so tall. But that's when I feel the seeds of an eating disorder were planted.

"When Leslie did develop anorexia, it was a devastating, helpless feeling; I thought there was a chance that, after visiting her at college and seeing how she looked . . . her father and I thought she might die. I remember unscrewing a jar of peanut butter we had bought for her when we set her up for the semester three months earlier and there was a tiny little divot in the top level of peanut butter. Like she had maybe touched her pinkie finger and then pulled away. It broke my heart.

"For me personally, being diagnosed with multiple sclerosis has been the biggest hurdle. I get angry. It's unbelievably frustrating to have your body not do what you want it to do. Oh, and talk about body image: Having to use a cane really does a number on you, because you associate canes with being much older, but all of a sudden it's something you have to depend on. But when other women who have just been diagnosed with MS ask me for advice, I say you have to use it, both for safety and so strangers don't think you're drunk! You have to have a sense of humor to help you along.

"I've gotten through all of this with acceptance and encouragement of friends and family, and with their patience. You have to get to the point where you get over it and accept yourself for what you are. You've gotta suck it up. I had to actually jab a huge needle into my thigh muscle a few times when my doctor was out of town and you know what? It stunk. So I lined up my Hershey's Kisses and unwrapped each one and ate about six of them, and then when I had a little sugar buzz, I pulled my jeans down and I did it. You have to concentrate on what you can do, not what you can't.

"Now, I'm much more aware of how physical issues affect girls of all ages—my young students who won't eat crackers because they don't want to be fat, the struggles young adults face like Les did, and now the battles of older people my age with medical problems. But I think in the long run, I've come out on top. There comes a point where you have to find and rely on an inner strength. It's like Leslie's grandfather always says, it doesn't matter how many times you fall, it's how many times you get back up. That's why my license plates says what it says: GT BK UP."

Becky, ninety-one, a yoga instructor:

"I've been teaching yoga since 1960. Before that, I taught third grade on Chicago's South Side for almost forty years, but I was always interested in yoga. I remember riding the school bus as a young girl and reading an article about it and it said if you wanted to teach yoga, you had to travel to India and get a guru and I started crying because I didn't think I'd ever get there. From that time on, I knew it would be something I would do. I think it was because I did yoga in another lifetime and wanted to continue in this life. I really do.

"As a younger girl, I didn't think about my body at all. It was only after I became involved with yoga that I truly started paying attention to my body. I changed my diet. I stopped eating meat. Why? I just felt it was not healthy for the body. I've only had one sip of coffee in my entire life—it smells so good but it made my mouth go like this [Becky makes a puckering face] and now I only have milk or tea. And no alcohol. I once had a drink of something and it made me dizzy, so I never touched it again.

"After I got into yoga, I started fasting and got slimmer and slimmer. I went on my first ten-day fast and felt so energetic, happy, and healthy. I've been fasting now for several years. But I drink water, of course. Distilled, never tap. I can read the phone book without reading glasses and I have never been sick, haven't had a cold or cough in forty years. I'm ninety-one years old but I've never been sick.

"Yoga helps you first get more in touch with your spirit, then comes the body. When I first began studying yoga, I was taking lessons by mail, and I thought yoga was entirely meditative. All I was doing was meditating. So when I went to California to study, to become initiated, I saw people in all of these poses, people doing shoulder-stands, upside down. I didn't even know there was a physical aspect of it. Now, I can do shoulder-stands, everything. In fact, when training, I had to do a hundred yogic push-ups, and I don't need to wear a bra anymore. [She begins to take her sweater off in the middle of the bookstore to prove it, but I stop her just after seeing the lower half of her right breast. She's right. No bra.] I would undress in front of any man, any man. I've worked with my body. There's no sagging under my arms, no sagging breasts. No hang-ups about this body.

"People usually don't believe it when they learn my age. They'll say, 'Are you really?' or 'I don't believe you. Show me your driver's license.'

"Let me tell you a story. I was at Marshall Fields the other day in the cosmetics section and the woman was trying to sell me eye cream. She said, 'You need to use this because when you get to be sixty, you'll start to develop wrinkles.' And I said, 'Lady, I'm ninety!' And she called all the women over and said, 'Look, this woman is ninety years old!' They couldn't believe it. They just couldn't believe it.

"I believe in focusing on the body, as long as we remember we are not the body; and if you focus too much on the body, you lose what you really are. And what you really are is a beautiful daughter of God. First, realize you are a spiritual soul. The body is a vessel. And that's what's wrong with the world today—we're so interested in the I, the me, that we don't realize we're more than the body. We're the mind and spirit. That's why I don't really consider myself an African American woman. Because I believe in reincarnation, I see myself as a Greek woman, an Egyptian woman. So I just think of myself as a citizen of the world, like Socrates.

"My advice to younger women would be to take care of your body by eating right, by not smoking, not drinking. Don't get overweight. Be sure you get enough omega 3 and flaxseed oil, that kind of thing. Vitamins and supplements. Yoga, definitely. But realize you are more than the body. You are the spirit and the body is just the clothing. If you focus on your spirit and your mind, your body will be radiant."

Epilogue:
Smokin' in the Girls' Room

Time to Throw in the Towel on Hating Our Bodies

So I'm feeling ready to return to the women's locker room as a participant, no longer the observer, the researcher, the gonzo journalist. After more than five years of asking questions, jotting notes, and basically acting like an all-around Peeping Tomassinna, I'm longing for the days when my post-workout routine consisted of a quick shower, maybe a steam, and a friendly chat with girlfriends, minus any conscious analysis or purposefully watchful eye.

In simpler words: I'm sick of staring at T & A.

But I fear my homecoming to the locker room might not go as smoothly as I might have hoped. I'll be like the retired dentist at a cocktail party, subconsciously eyeing guests' teeth, thinking, "Hmmm, I wonder whether he knows about the new laser whitening treatments?" It's difficult to stop caring about a subject you once immersed yourself in; nearly impossible to erase the passion you once felt for a topic. And so I suspect I will continue to hear women's digs and insults rise above the din of the locker room chatter, will still watch that damn Toledo scale like a ladyhawk.

And all things considered, that's okay. It's an incredible tradeoff for the number of positive changes I've already witnessed in my life, just in the time it took to write this baby. Each one has been a direct result of speaking with the women in this book. The honesty in their comments and their brave willingness to mine with me the emotional bomb-riddled territory that is body image, regardless of whether I was a close friend or a total stranger, is to be applauded.

The transformations in my life have been as subtle as the scent of the vanilla lotion my sister, Jessica, applies after her workouts, but as far-reaching as the fifty-mile walk my other sister, Sarah, and I recently slogged through to raise money for multiple sclerosis research. For instance, I'm now a bit more cognizant of the impact my walking around topless in the locker room can have. From the Thoroughly Modest Millies to the culturally reserved women working on staff, I realized it wasn't worth *that* much to me to make others squirm.

Now don't get me wrong—I in no way support the "No Nudity" policies that dictate behavior in certain locker rooms. I still blow-dry topless at the vanity if I'm in a hurry. I just make more of an effort to cover up Poncho and Lefty (as Pamela Anderson so eloquently calls hers) if I'm spending more than a few minutes there. Kind of like a "Do Unto Others" thing. I even found myself watching once as another woman slowly and meticulously applied her makeup, breasts breathing easy. It felt to me that if she was a TV news show, the ticker at the bottom would be scrolling, "Look at me.

Look at me. Please look at me." It made me wonder, "Huh, I wonder what she's trying to prove?"

Another major change came when, for quite possibly the first time since I began to crawl, I didn't work out on my birthday. Like many women I spoke with, I've always exercised extra diligently on my birthday because I know I'll be going to a nice restaurant and will want to indulge, and also because it makes me feel good about myself and how I look. But this year, I was busy writing at a coffee shop, and then I spent some time napping. Looking back on my calendar, there's nothing written down, so it's not as if I had any plans to preclude me from an endorphin-boosting five-mile run. I think it was a combination of dedication to the book, an increased comfort level with my body, and maybe a self-dare; a challenge to see whether I could do it, if I could break the chain.

And I did. I also showered at home instead of the gym—something I hardly ever do—and was whisked away to a hip Asian fusion restaurant where a surprise party awaited me. I ordered a mango martini (okay, three) and downed a delicious beef-with-mushroom dish. And I felt beautiful the whole evening long.

Then there was the baby scream that I thought would never happen. No, it's not what you think. One day my manager, Kristin, called me into her office to share some important news. My mind raced. Was I being put on probation for Googling "girls" and "locker room"? Because I swear, that is not some sort of pervert fetish of mine. It was for research and besides, I was on my lunch break.

"I wanted to let you know, I'm going to have a baby," Kristin said to me from behind her desk with her trademark degree of measured calmness. The words didn't hit me immediately—they just kind of hung in the air, like humidity. Our friend and coworker Debbie had just come racing over—I now know it was because she wanted to see my reaction. You know, ha ha, let's shock Leslie into heart-attack mode and watch as she tries to cover her pregnancy anxiety and fear of losing her favorite boss ever with a hearty *Mazel Tov*. But I swear on Kristin's 36 EE maternity bra of biblical proportions that, once the news sunk in, I shrieked with such absolute unadulterated joy that even I was surprised. I was jumping up and down, running around her office, practically crying tears of happiness. From where was this reaction coming?

Upon further thought, I realized it was just weeks before that I had performed my Empathy Belly experiment. Could fifteen cups of fake amniotic fluid and a metal tap-dancing bladder ball have made that much of a difference? Then I remembered Kristin had asked me all sorts of questions about what it had been like wearing the vest: How did it feel? Was I sore afterward? Surely, she had known she was preggers at that time. And *she* was picking *my* brain! I realized my excitement came from a certain connection I felt I would never have experienced if I had not gotten the chance to be "pregnant." So although I'm not ready to go shopping for a baby jogger just yet, my perspective on motherhood did change. And thus, the student had become the teacher.

But perhaps the best teachers were those seniors who shared their stories. One woman whose story really stuck with me is Harriet, the PR exec, who described body image as an ongoing thorn in her side since before puberty. Having been teased by some kids about her "piano legs" left a lasting scar on her body image, rendering exercise an obsession for nearly her entire life.

Like Harriet, I was teased when I was younger for being chubby, when actually I had a hypothyroid condition. As soon as my magical blue pills kicked in, I shot up about a foot while remaining the same weight. But so help me God, I will never forget being called a "cow" in fourth grade by a certain young man who shall remain nameless (Matt). That label stayed with me, glued to my back like a Kick Me sign, just as "piano legs" stayed with Harriet. And, like her, as a result of that stupid comment, I saw myself as being very fat. And sometimes I *still* have to struggle, decades later, to remember I'm not.

Harriet spoke of looking back at a picture of herself as a young girl and marveling at all of the life decisions she's made based on her fear of gaining weight. I don't want that to happen to me—it's already happened enough times. So I've made it a point to sit Harriet on my shoulder and carry her with me, drawing strength from her words at times when I need them most.

I've also enjoyed seeing the effect this book has had on those around me. By that I mean most women and men who know I've been researching body image through the lens of the locker room have become more sensitive to the issue, their eyes and ears opened to issues that may previously have gone unnoticed.

One of my favorites was when my father-in-law, a six-foot-two lawyer with a rather imposing presence, called me from his cell phone to tell me about a song he had just heard on the radio called "Tiny Heinie Girl" by artist Bayne Gibby.

"It's all about this girl who's waiting in line for the showers in the locker room and the girl in front of her has a smaller butt than she does!" Peter practically giggled to me, obviously proud of his discovery. "You should look it up. It's 'Tiny Heinie—H-E-I-N-I-E—Girl.'"

No, hysterical is what it was.

Another example: Come summertime, when college kids returned from campus for a few months, our gym filled up with coeds. One of them was a young woman suffering from severe anorexia, probably quite similar in appearance to how I looked my freshman year when I came home. I hadn't seen her, but many of my gym friends had and oh, how they clamored to inform me of her presence. Some even tried to nail down her schedule so that I could "catch" her for an interview. Again, the book's message was hard at work, raising people's awareness.

Finally, and one story that still brings a smile to my face every time I think about it: Debbie, who verbally whupped me for letting my boobs hang out in the locker room, admitted she was trying a little experiment of her own, attempting to reveal more of *her* ta-tas, bit by bit, in the locker room. It was challenging, she confessed, so I gave her some pointers, such as maybe just letting one breast peek out on her way to the shower, or hiking her towel up to just below the bra-line, but obscuring her nakedness with her shampoo and conditioner bottles. As she got more comfortable, she could try easing her way into full topless mode. Baby steps.

The Ultimate Cool-Down

For anyone who has ever taken yoga, I think you'll agree that the best part is the end, when the instructor turns the lights down low and instructs you to lie back, close your eyes, and relax every muscle in your body. Called, rather morbidly, Corpse Pose (why can't they go with something more upbeat, such as Sunshine Acceptance? After all, this is the same position I assume while lying out in the sun), this is the time to bring balance and relaxation to every cell of your body, explained Becky, the ninety-one-year-old yoga instructor. "You're getting rid of worry and anxiety and stress," Becky said. The purpose is to clear the mind, "to forget about the I, me, and mine and go to your soul." In other words, this is not the time for heavy mental lifting. Not the time to worry about what you're going to pick up for dinner, how many meetings you have at work tomorrow, how your thighs look while splayed out on the yoga mat.

And so I ask you to clear your mind and recall my initial plea from the introduction of this book. I spoke passionately of the need to tame the inner demon that paralyzes so many of us into a state of broken body image—to slaughter the demons that cause us to greet ourselves in the mirror, not with admiration, but with "whys" and "if-onlys." *Why* am I so fat? *Why* don't I look like the model in the magazine? *If only* my thighs were like those of the woman on the Stairmaster next to me and didn't touch.

It is my hope—my low-fat, pie-in-the-sky locker room dream—that after reading this book you will be able to cross at least one "if-only" off your list. I'm not expecting women everywhere to smash their scales, shed their insecurities, and sail through life unburdened by body-image woes. (Although wouldn't a mass scale-smashing be amazing? Kind of like a modern-day bra burning?) But I'd like to think I'm not just toiling aimlessly in an effort to empty sand from the ocean of unhealthy self-image. As Dr. Zager, the psychologist who works with young women, put it, "Eventually, there could be a critical mass." It's up to us women—from inside the locker room and out—to band together and, as I've said before, screw the scale and live large, no matter what we weigh. And when that happens, can you imagine the freedom that will come by liberating ourselves from the body-image albatross that has been chained around our necks—and our psyches— like a sweaty, moldy gym towel for all of these years? It will be revolutionary, I swear on my purple yoga sticky mat.

Brick by Brick

I find it incredibly ironic that just as I finish up this book, my gym is in the midst of renovating the women's locker room. Chunky tiles in shades of royal cobalt and buttery yellow line the shower stalls, replacing the smaller, neutral-colored squares forever lined in white caulk; new granite counter- tops shimmer when the overhead light bounces off them. The white plastic soap and body shampoo pumps have been replaced with polished silver, and they dispense just the right amount of product with the slightest touch. A flat- screen television and computers have even been installed, fi- nally putting us on par with the men.

It's so ironic that just as I'm about to leave my locker room, metaphorically speaking, it's having new life breathed into it. Maybe my endless months of interviewing and searching have been subconsciously noticed by the health club staff and they've decided to step it up a notch. Or, in a more magical land, perhaps the walls have witnessed and heard the same anecdotes I've jotted down in my diary, and they've cried out for the type of space we ladies deserve. Or, and I suppose this is the most realistic, it just has to do with the fact that we're under new management and they're finally making some much-needed changes. Anyhow, I hope I haven't freaked out club members with my tales of sock-footed shower romping and steam-room gossip listening. I'd like to stick around and enjoy the revamped space. It should be beautiful.

Speaking of paying renewed attention to our surroundings, the other day I attended a book reading by the author and fellow gym-goer Rob Sullivan, who asked the audience to do an exercise based on the Law of Attraction. He had everyone look around the coffee shop we were in and try to memorize everything red we could see. My eyes darted around the room from a painting on the wall to my toenail polish to the dress of a woman sitting by the window to a box of passion fruit teabags for sale near the café. As I tried to commit all things ruby to memory, he asked us to close our eyes.

"Now," he said, "try to think of everything in the room that's yellow."

We all laughed because the task was impossible—as he explained, we train ourselves to see what we want to see. Now, I realize that if I start to pay attention and listen for positive comments or experiences in the locker room, if I look for the yellow and not the red, I might just luck out and unearth a body-image gem. Such as when, a few months ago, two girls, maybe ten years old or so, were goofing off as their mother got dressed after her shower. They experimented with hair sprays and deodorants, primped in the mirror, tried to squeeze into the lockers and hide from one another. Eventually, their exploits led them to . . . yep, you guessed it. The scale. As I blow-dried my hair, I leaned back to watch as each of them hopped on and watched the needle make its way toward nine o'clock.

When their mother was ready, she called the girls and they darted away from the scale, one after the other. As each of them slung their gym bags over their shoulders, the taller girl called out, at full volume, "Guess what, Mom? I weigh 78 pounds. Isn't that great?" Not a drop of concern—or pride, for that matter—in her voice. Just a matter of fact.

And as the trio rounded the corner to exit our locker room, I saw it: the yellow. The mother rubbed the back of her young daughter—not yet burdened by issues of weight and body image—and smiled as she confirmed, "It sure is, Kiddo. You should definitely be proud—of every last ounce of it."

Acknowledgments

First, and foremost, I need to thank my beautiful and talented publicist friend Michelle Aielli, who called me up one day and asked, "Have you ever thought about writing a book?" Because that happens. In addition to introducing me to The Man Who Would Become My Agent, Larry Weissman, Michelle has stood by me every step of the way, serving as reader, brainstormer, and one-woman support system. Thank you, Michelle. You are a true gem.

Thank you to Larry, who helped turn *Locker Room Diaries* from a leopard-print journal into what you hold in your hands today. You ushered me through the process with style and strength and for that, I am grateful. I will always think of you when I am in the locker room, surrounded by women in various stages of undress. You are welcome.

Team Da Capo—Marnie Cochran, Wendy Holt, Kate Kazeniac, Bill Smith, Erin Sprague, and Jennifer Blakebrough-Raeburn—one thousand thank yous for your support for and belief in this project. Wendy, it has been an exceptional pleasure working with you . . . and by "working with" I mean your ability to juggle my emails and assuage my often semi-frantic phone calls with your gentle, reassuring voice, all while serving as a fabulous editor and teacher.

Thank you to all of the women who bared their souls for this book.

To Kristin Reynolds and Catharine Hamrick, my eternal gratitude for making it possible for me to write this book . . . and you know what I mean. Kristin, especially, thank you for serving as the most wonderfully inspiring mentor a young writer could ask for.

Much love and appreciation to my family for always believing in me, particularly my incredible parents, Donna and Jerry Goldman, and grandparents Jean and Mort Schur. Love also to Peter and Barbra Alter and Papa Bob Goldman. To my brother, Jeff: Your never-give-up attitude has served as an incredible inspiration. Don't think all those nights you stayed up until 3:00 a.m. pumping out screenplays in high school went unnoticed, Jinky.

Jan Deadman of Madison East High School, thank you for helping me get pregnant for a day, when nobody else would.

Love to my caring friends, particularly those who have always been supportive of my writing: Laura Baranowski, Lauren Brody, Debbie Broutman, Jill Butensky, Trish Figueroa, Dave Fogelson, Diane Hepps, Elizabeth Kerr, Randi Klebanoff, Amanda Nelson, Alicia Newland, Kate Phair, Julie Smolyansky, Eden Shaffer, Alison Sadowy, Chuck Sanchez, Susie Sondag, Heidi Tarr, and Veronica Vasquez. Eternal thanks to those who helped me plant my feet in the writing field: Al Gunther, Melanie Mannarino, Duane Swierczynski, and Ross Werland.

And to my tremendous husband, Dan: You not only put up with two years of conversations that began, "So, Leslie, I hear you're writing a book . . . ," you championed it. You listened to endless locker room stories and picked me up from the gym a bazillion times without complaint. You were there for me during every near meltdown, writing related or otherwise. You are my human Paxil . . . and my best friend. Thank you. I love you.